Team Dentistry

Chairside procedures and
practice management

For my wife Jennifer, my children Jonathan,
Alexis, Benjamin and Gideon and in
memory of my late parents.

Clinical Techniques in Dentistry

Team Dentistry

Chairside procedures and practice management

J Ellis Paul

BDS, LDS, VU(Manc)

MARTIN DUNITZ

© J Ellis Paul 1991

First published in the United Kingdom in 1991 by Martin Dunitz Ltd, 7–9 Pratt Street, London NW1 0AE

British Library Cataloguing-in-Publication Data
Paul, J Ellis
   Team dentistry
   1. Dentistry
   I. Title   II. Series
   617.6
   ISBN 0-948269-78-2

Publisher's note

Information on cross-infection control is given according to guidelines current for Europe and the USA at the time of going to press. The latest guidelines, obtained from the relevant authority, should always be consulted.

Photoset by Scribe Design, Gillingham, Kent
Originated, printed and bound in Singapore by Toppan Co (S) Pte Ltd

Contents

Preface   vii

Acknowledgments   viii

Sources   viii

Part I Practice management

1 Practice image   3

2 Marketing dentistry—the practice builder   11

3 Time management   29

4 Financial control   45

5 Computers in dental practice   53
   Anthony S Kravitz, BDS

Part II Team dentistry

6 Working in the seated posture   69

7 Maintenance of correct posture   78

8 Efficient utilization of the dental assistant   88

9 Maintenance of a clear operating field   96

10 Maintenance of operating vision   106

11 Instrument handling   116

12 Cross-infection control   135

13 Work simplification   149

Part III Applications to clinical procedures

14 Preparatory procedures   157

15 Restorative procedures—amalgam   168

16 Restorative procedures—composites   177

17 Prosthodontic procedures   184

18 Endodontic procedures   203

19 Teaching four-handed dentistry   206

Reading list   209

Index   211

Preface

After 20 years of postgraduate teaching of practice management and four-handed dentistry, it has become increasingly apparent to me that there is a need for a practice text which, though primarily dealing with clinical aspects of team dentistry, also includes the most important areas of practice management which directly relate to this.

In attempting to meet this need, I hope that I have produced in one volume a thorough guide to smoother and more efficient practice both inside and outside the treatment area. This book is chiefly for the dentist in general practice. The emphasis throughout is on the practical aspects and it is aimed not just at the dentist but also at the entire dental team, including the dental assistant and the receptionist. It is hoped that it will also be of value to the dental student and trainee dental assistant.

All the techniques shown in the book are based on those which I have developed and refined in over 20 years of research and teaching of the subject throughout the world and which I have found most successful in my own general practice. I hope the reader will study them with an open mind and at least try to be objective in using any new ideas. Much of the first section dealing with practice management is based on the highly successful series of seminars on the subject which my colleague Barry Posner BDS and I have given for over 10 years throughout the UK. I have limited the contents of this section only to the areas which our experience clearly showed were those which gave general dental practitioners most problems and on which they needed guidance. It is not intended to be a comprehensive text on practice management. There is a plethora of books dealing purely with this aspect in far greater detail. This book is designed rather to solve many of the day-to-day problems in general practice and so to contribute to a reduction in the level of stress and an increase in practice efficiency. Similarly, the chapter on cross-infection control is not intended as an exhaustive reference, but as a set of straightforward guidelines for use in daily practice.

All the photographs, other than those where a source is acknowledged, were taken by the author not in a studio but deliberately in the more natural environment of his own practice. Though the former might have produced photography of a higher quality, it is felt that readers would be able to relate more to an actual working treatment area.

The use throughout the text of the masculine pronoun for patient and dentist, and the feminine for dental assistant, is purely in the interest of brevity. I fully appreciate that patients, dentists and dental assistants may be either male or female. Also, for the sake of brevity, the initials DA have been used to denote dental assistant.

It is hoped that this book will show all progressive dentists, regardless of country, how to deliver a high standard of dental care, with efficiency but without stress. Improving standards in clinical practice through organization and efficiency will leave the entire dental team happier and more satisfied.

JEP

Acknowledgments

A great number of people have been of considerable assistance in both the preparation and production of this book. I should like to express my thanks to the following:

Peter Galgut who first proposed the idea of my writing it and who subsequently gave me a great deal of time and advice in suggesting improvements to the text.

Lucy Hamilton of Martin Dunitz for all her time and expertise in editing the book, Mary Banks for her many helpful suggestions and Celia Caspell for copy-editing the final text.

My loyal secretary, Philomena Whelan, for typing the whole of the first draft and to Bernie Griffiths for her expertise and many hours of work in the typing of the second and final draft.

My dental assistants, Claire Robertson, Pamela Howard, Emma Towey and Denise Walker, for their help and patience during many hours of photography.

My two young colleagues, Lynn Goldwater BDS and Nigel Day BDS, for their skill and patience while acting as dentists for many of the photographs.

My colleague, Philip Wander BDS, for helping me to become a better photographer.

Professor PF Harris, Department of Anatomy, University of Manchester, for his help with Chapter 6.

Bernard Sylvester FRCS, consultant orthopaedic surgeon, for his helpful comments on Chapters 6 and 7.

Dr JL Altshuler, Boston, for his many very positive and helpful suggestions for text improvements.

Dr Michael Martin, University of Liverpool, for his guidance and many useful suggestions and comments on Chapter 12.

Glover Dental Supplies, J & S Davies, Wright Health Group, Sycom Ltd and A Davis of Safeguard Systems for the loan of material and equipment.

And finally my dear wife Jennifer, truly a woman of worth, for her many helpful suggestions, constant encouragement and support.

Sources

The author wishes to thank A Lockyer for Figure 2.1, PA Wander for Figure 2.2 and PF Harris for Figures 6.5–6.6. Figure 16.15 is reproduced by permission of *The Dentist* and Figures 6.11–6.13 by that of *Dental Practice*. Figures 6.2–6.4, 6.10 and 7.3 are adapted from illustrations in *Home Position Perception and Movements in Dentistry*, Shoji Y (MDP: Tokyo 1974). Figure 7.2 is adapted from material supplied by J Morita Corporation, Tokyo. Figure 11.1 is adapted from *A Practical Guide to Assisted Operating*, Paul JE (BDA: London 1972).

Part I Practice management

Practice image

1

In a world where the demand for dental treatment is falling and the number of dentists increasing, more positive efforts must be made to attract patients to dental practices. To this end, one of the more important factors is the presentation of a good practice image. An attractive and distinctive image, displaying character and good taste, will make a practice stand out from others in the area and will have a very positive effect on increasing patient numbers. Moreover a modern appearance implies a progressive dentist practising all the latest techniques—a factor which is also likely to attract new patients. With the increasing significance of cosmetic dentistry, an aesthetic image is all-important. There are two other advantages:

● A pleasant and relaxing decor has a great effect in the reduction of patient apprehension (Paul, 1976). The total ambience of the practice must make it welcoming and non-threatening.
● A pleasing working environment raises the level of morale and therefore of performance of all members of staff (Paul and Posner, 1987).

The overall image must project to patients a relaxing, friendly atmosphere, a modern dentist and a happy, satisfied, well-motivated staff.

External decor

Good practice image starts at the entrance to the premises, so attention must be paid to the outside appearance. After all, this is the first feature of the practice that the incoming patient will see. The external appearance of the building must be clean, tidy, attractive and welcoming. It is important for the practice to be clearly visible. For example, premises painted pure white, and regularly maintained in order to keep the appearance fresh, will make a practice stand out and at the same time will project a very attractive, positive image which will draw patients to it. This outside factor is often overlooked by the rental tenant.

The front entrance is the first indirect contact the patient has with the dentist. The front door itself must therefore look clean and attractive. If it is unimpressive, consideration should be given to replacing the front entrance door with one from the wide range of attractive yet inexpensive doors freely available. However, often a coat of paint, new door accessories and a planted shrub in a suitably matching pot outside the entrance may be all that is needed to enhance the outward appearance and look attractive.

Internal decor

Internal decor can be broadly grouped into five categories:

● Textures
● Colours
● Lighting
● Windows
● Visual foci

Textures

Walls

Paint

This is perhaps the most widely used. It should always be matt finished rather than gloss. The latter tends to give a dated look to the room and appears too cold and clinical. The colour used is important and more will be said about this later in the chapter.

Paper

This provides an acceptable texture and has the advantage of being available in a wide range of colours, textures and patterns. Care must be taken to avoid patterns and colours which are too vivid and therefore not restful. A wide range of washable papers is now available, with the obvious advantage of being easily cleaned without the need to redecorate.

As an alternative to patterned papers, textured finishes, for example anaglypta, can be used. These can be painted over, giving both a coloured and textured wall finish. They have the advantage of providing a surface which is visually interesting and looks warm and relaxing.

Fabric wall-covering

Different fabrics and weaves of hessian (US: burlap) and other materials can be combined in the same room, using either different patterns and colours of the same material or different textures of the same colour. They do not necessarily have to be used on all four walls of the room but can be combined by using, for example, hessian or fabric on one or two walls and paint on the remainder.

Cork

This can be obtained in either sheet or tile form. Again it provides both a warm colour and texture, but its use should be limited to one wall because the very rich texture can tend to dominate the room.

Wood

This is available in a wide variety of grains, widths and colours. It can be stained or varnished to provide both an attractive colour and a warm texture. It is very modern and clean-looking but, like cork, should be limited to one wall if it is not to become too dominating a texture. It also has the advantage of providing a pleasing background for highly coloured wall-hangings, pictures or sculptures. Wood can be used very effectively as a facing to an existing painted wall. It should be lightly coloured and preferably of an open structure so that it does not become too dominant and does not obscure the colour of the wall underneath.

Natural brick

This obviously can only be used within custom-built premises and should also be used in moderation.

Too much brick is cold and uninviting, but, if confined to one or two walls, it provides a pleasant contrast to more conventional textures. The most pleasing appearance is achieved by the use of rough-surface bricks and these can be obtained in a wide range of colours and textures.

Although the last four materials are initially more costly, they are durable and therefore most economical in the long term, since the need for redecorating is much reduced.

Because all six types of materials are used domestically, they are familiar to patients and produce a warm, soft environment which is pleasing to the eye. Where the texture or colour is neutral, it should be used to provide a suitable background on which to hang brightly coloured pictures or photographs, perhaps taken by the dentist, to enhance this effect. Local art dealers are often willing to lend framed prints and paintings to be hung in the practice in return for displaying the dealer's name and address. The advantage is that, apart from being free of charge, the paintings can be changed periodically.

Floors

Carpet is recommended in all non-clinical areas. Its use makes it far easier to achieve a warm, relaxed environment.

In the treatment area, vinyl, wood or parquet flooring must be used around the immediate chairside area for reasons of cleanliness and sterility. In the non-chairside areas, carpet should be used since it helps to subdue the cold, clinical effect. However, it should not be of the deep-pile variety because this tends to act as a dust and debris collector and is difficult to clean to an adequate standard of hygiene. Where carpet is used in the treatment area, it should be of densely packed synthetic fibre, preferably stain-resistant and easily cleaned.

Ceilings

As most dentists now work in a seated position by the side of a supine patient, it is important to remember that during treatment the patient probably sees the ceiling for a far greater proportion of the time than he does the rest of the treatment area. Particular care must therefore be taken in the way the ceiling is finished. In older buildings, rooms often have high ceilings with attractive decorative features. These should not be eliminated but rather emphasized by careful use of colour. Attractive mouldings can be picked out and highlighted by painting them in a contrasting colour. Where the ceiling is high but not aesthetically attractive, it can be painted out in a very dark colour and suspended lighting used to throw light down and away from it. However, ideally a suspended ceiling using acoustic tiles should be fitted. This looks modern and is pleasing to the eye. It has the added advantage of permitting light fittings to be recessed and gives a high level of light reflection.

It is helpful to provide focal points on which the supine patient can concentrate. This serves to divert attention from the treatment being given and makes the patient less apprehensive. For example small mobiles can be suspended from the ceiling (this is particularly good for children) or an attractive focus of attention provided by a ceiling mural or by a very large photograph mounted onto the ceiling directly in the eye-line of the supine patient. This should preferably be on a colourful, attractive and restful theme and contain a large amount of detail which requires patient concentration. For example several dentists have a large aerial photograph of a section of their city. This gives a very good focus of attention because the patient can try to identify familiar landmarks and streets.

Colours

Correct selection of colour is perhaps the most important factor in establishing the right image of the environment. It also has a proven psychological effect on patients and staff. The right colour can soothe, relax and reassure the patient; a bad choice may excite, stimulate or irritate him.

Colour schemes can be either monochromatic or complementary.

Monochromatic colour schemes

These can be either the same shade or different shades of the same colour. Used alone, this type of scheme can sometimes appear monotonous, so small areas of contrasting colour and textures could be added.

Complementary or harmonious colour schemes

These schemes involve the use of closely related colours. Bright red should be avoided, particularly in the waiting area, since it implies danger, heat and irritation. Where red is used, it should tend more towards maroon or orange, both of which are warmer and richer, and therefore do not irritate. Either of these shades provides a warm contrast to more neutral colours and textures.

In general, colours from the middle of the spectrum should be used such as yellow, orange, brown, beige and green. Yellow and orange are the colours of sunshine and therefore are warm and comforting, while brown, beige and green are colours associated with trees, grass and plants and so are familiar and reassuring. Blue is a difficult colour to use because it must be exactly the right shade. Too deep a shade is depressing and can make the room appear small; too light a shade, such as ice-blue, is cold and cheerless. Grey and mauve are usually associated with dignity and professionalism.

Derivatives of all the above colours in pale pastel shades are found to be the most acceptable and are both relaxing and cheerful.

In the treatment area the problem of colour choice is slightly different. More than ever before, it is important to convey a message of cleanliness and sterility. Though an all-white room would successfully convey this message, it would look too clinical and cold. The best solution is either to use very pale pastel shades, which help the room to look warmer, or to use white as a background to large areas of bright colour and accessory decorative items such as pictures, fabric hangings, sculptures and reliefs. Alternatively, colour can be introduced through equipment and cabinetry. White or very pale walls around colour-strong equipment will convey the right image of cleanliness without the overall effect being too clinical and cold.

Lighting

The most important factors when assessing the lighting conditions for the dental practice are illuminance, luminance distribution, the reflection of light, and colour rendering.

- *Illuminance* is the amount of light per unit area and is measured in lux (1 lumen/m^2).
- *Luminance* expresses the intensity of light emitted.
- The *reflection factor* measures the amount of light reflected from a surface compared with the amount of light reflected from a perfectly matt, white surface, under conditions of equal source intensity.
- The *colour-rendering index* (R_a) measures the ability of a light source to reproduce a colour on a scale of 0–100. Thus a light source with a good colour rendering has an R_a index of over 90.

The work of the dental team is demanding, not only physically but also visually, because of the need to work very precisely on a small and detailed area. Unsatisfactory lighting conditions can cause mental and physical fatigue and in particular contribute to poor posture; however, most importantly, the quality of work can be affected. Since details of a task are seen more easily as illuminance increases, it is therefore extremely important that both the ambient lighting of the treatment area and the localized intensive lighting of the mouth are of the highest order of illuminance. That around the dental chair should be at least 4000 lux and that on the patient's face not less than 15 000 lux.

Glare

Glare leads to discomfort and a reduction of the ability to see objects. It can be caused by having too high a luminance – because of direct light from bright indoor lighting or the sun – or too high a reflection factor from glossy surfaces. For this reason, all light sources should be screened with some form of baffle or louvre and all surfaces should be non-glossy wherever possible.

Forms of lighting

Other than the operating light itself, there are basically three types of lighting required for the practice:

- Functional
- Background
- Decor

Functional lighting

In the treatment area, a high level of ambient lighting is required and the relation between the illumination of the mouth and that of the surroundings should be 4:1. This can only be provided by siting directly over the chair and working surfaces fluorescent tubes with illuminance of not less than 1000 lux each, to provide a total illuminance of 4000 lux. However, the lights must always be covered by some form of louvre and must be recessed into the ceiling wherever possible. This is one of the advantages of using a suspended ceiling.

The type of fluorescent tube used in the treatment area is most important—particularly for shade matching. Colour-corrected fluorescent tubes should be used. North-light colour matching is closest to north sky light and therefore best for the critical judgment of shades.

There are now several types of fluorescent fittings designed specifically for working environments. These have tubes of high luminous efficiency and a good colour-rendering index resembling that of daylight. They have extra dazzle protection provided by special specular louvres which are highly polished. Together with the parabolic form of the reflector they provide excellent optical control and luminous efficiency. Other advantages of these systems are reduced power consumption, low heat output and noise levels, and elimination of stroboscopic effects.

Though fluorescent lighting in the treatment area is the most important, it should be softened by the additional use of small tungsten spotlights, which can be used to highlight decorative features such as plants, pictures or sculptures.

Outside the treatment area, tungsten lighting of 300–400 lux should be used since this is not as harsh as fluorescent lighting and is more warm and relaxing.

Background lighting

This should be of the tungsten variety and should be used in reception, waiting and administrative areas. In the last, a high level of ambient lighting is required and this can easily be achieved by the use of suitable tungsten lights of high illuminance or the use of reflector bulbs. Low voltage bulbs provide high illumination with low energy consumption. The waiting room should be the most relaxing room in the practice, to minimize patient apprehension. To this end, the lighting should be bright enough to read by but not so bright that it induces glare. Ideally, individual lights should be provided for each chair and these can be ceiling, wall-mounted or free-standing standard lamps. Whatever type of lighting is used, it should be well shaded to reduce glare.

Decor lighting

This complements the background lighting and takes the form of small spotlights which illuminate decorative features such as paintings, plants or sculptures. Fluorescent lights can be used provided they are hidden from direct view by a shade. This is particularly important in the waiting room where possibly only the smaller or architectural tubes should be utilized.

Windows

Window frames should be well maintained and kept scrupulously clean. All windows should be covered with some form of curtains or blinds to ensure privacy and soften the cold, impersonal look which bare windows give. A pleasant view from the window should not be obscured. In this case, net curtains will be sufficient both to provide privacy and to remove the starkness of the windows. This softening effect can be further enhanced by a pelmet and mock drapes. Though some authorities feel these are unacceptable in the treatment areas on hygienic grounds, they can certainly be used in the waiting, reception and consulting areas to provide a decorative feature. Alternatively, vertical louvre linen blinds can be used. These look modern and attractive and can be opened sufficiently to allow some natural daylight in. They also have the advantage of being flame-proof. Vertical louvre blinds are obtainable in a wide range of colours and in two widths of slats. A suitable colour and width

should be selected to blend with the overall decor. They should be cleaned periodically

Venetian blinds are becoming increasingly unpopular since they look unattractive, retain dust and debris, and are very difficult to clean.

Where the view from the window is unattractive, the window should be covered with either thicker net curtains or fine-textured, light-coloured vertical blinds which are kept closed. In both cases, these obscure the view while allowing in natural light.

Visual foci

These are distinctive and non-clinical features to which the patient's attention is drawn on first entering the treatment area. A strategically placed object such as a decorative plant arrangement, sculpture, aquarium or painting should be the first feature seen by the patient entering the room. It provides a non-dental focal point and will draw his attention away from what he dislikes most—the dental unit. This can be another facet in the overall reduction of patient apprehension.

Music

Though not classified as decor, background music is certainly a part of the dental environment and makes an important contribution to practice image. It is increasingly used in dental practice because it distracts the patients' attention, and helps them to relax, so reducing apprehension. Music can be provided either by a generalized system, for all patients and staff, or by a personal system, for the patient undergoing treatment.

Generalized system

This relays music from a central source to every room. Its advantage is that the entire practice can be supplied from the same source. The type of music must be carefully chosen and should be relaxing, unobtrusive and at a low level. It must be emphasized that excessive noise can have a counterproductive effect and even cause irritation. The type of music unit should also be carefully chosen and must not require constant attention by members of staff. Various machines are available which will play consecutive tapes for long periods of time without attention. There are also audio systems, complete with tapes, supplied and maintained by commercial firms and these have the advantage of using music professionally selected to fulfil all the necessary criteria.

Personal system

As an alternative to a generalized music system, a more local form of music can be provided by a small tape player with headphones worn by the patient. Its advantage is that only the patient can hear the music. Its disadvantage is that it is confined to the treatment area and cannot be heard in the reception and waiting areas. The type of headphones chosen is very important. Large headphones will impinge into the dentist's working area, interfere with the correct placement of his hands and cause him to work in a distorted posture. This can be avoided by using very small headphones such as those supplied with conventional personal stereo systems.

Control of temperature

The air temperature throughout the building must always be maintained at a comfortable level. Excessive heat or cold detracts from patient comfort and affects performance of dentists and staff. All central heating radiators should be unobtrusive while still being effective. Unsightly radiators should be obscured. A simple yet effective screen can be made from expanded aluminium mesh on a simple wood frame.

Air conditioning

In countries with temperate climates, too few dentists realize the importance of having the correct temperature constantly maintained throughout the practice by the use of air conditioning. This can be localized in the treatment areas (which tend to get hottest) but ideally it should be provided from a central source throughout every room. This requires ducting from the cooling source and can be costly and difficult to install in an existing building. It is much less costly to incorporate this type of system into custom-built premises. An ideal compromise is to position a single unit in every room which requires air conditioning. Such units are simple to install into an outside wall or window and can also incorporate heaters for use in the winter. Where wall or window installation is impractical, free-standing units are available.

Reception and waiting areas

Though the main purpose of this chapter is to discuss decor in general terms, there are several aspects specific to these two areas which should also be highlighted.

Reception

The receptionist is the patient's first human contact with the practice. The reception area must therefore project the correct image of warmth, care and quality. The reception desk or counter must look attractive, tidy and aesthetic. A high upstand to its front will very effectively screen the storage shelves and pigeon-holes necessary for efficient administration, and at the same time provide a surface of correct height for the patient to write on. The use of a closed-in reception desk with a sliding glass panel should be avoided completely since it gives the patient an impression of detachment and lack of personal contact. A smiling receptionist should be the first sight to greet patients when they enter.

Waiting area

The waiting area should have a number of functions besides that of occupying patients who are awaiting treatment. It should welcome patients, project the image of the practice, reduce apprehension and offer information about the services the practice offers. It can be either open plan, with a direct connection with the reception area, or a separate room. In either case, careful attention must be paid to decor and lighting and to the seating. Colours and textures must be warm and relaxing; lighting must be relaxing yet bright enough to read by and confined to tungsten lights. Seating should be comfortable and chairs arranged in very small groups. Rows of seats must be avoided where possible. The seating can also be used to introduce additional texture and colour.

Distractions should be provided such as background music, fish tanks, floral displays and attractive pictures. Photographs of the dentist's own personal interests and hobbies help to build a picture of the dentist as a human being. Many dentists like to display framed certificates of degrees, diplomas and advanced postgraduate courses attended. They feel that these enhance their professional reputation with the patients. However, such certificates must not dominate the waiting area.

Waiting time should be turned to advantage and the opportunity to use this time for positive dental education should not be neglected. Magazines should be few and up-to-date, and limited to those of a general nature rather than the glossy type of magazines such as travel, motoring and high fashion ones which may divert the patients' disposable income away from dentistry. They should be placed on a wall-mounted rack rather than on a table because this helps to keep them much tidier. The presence of dental educational material may also help to reduce apprehension by making dentistry approachable. However, like the magazines, such material must be carefully selected and discreetly displayed and limited in amount so that it will not detract from the restful, homely atmosphere the dentist has sought so carefully to create.

A video playing continuously provides not only a distraction but is also an excellent method of patient education. The necessity to leave practice portfolios and education material in the waiting area will be referred to in Chapter 2.

Children's corner

Whether the practice has a large or small percentage of children as patients, their special needs should be considered. This is especially important in the waiting area. Children are often even more apprehensive than adults, are easily bored and quickly become tense and fractious. This must be prevented by providing facilities to divert their attention during the time they are waiting. This can easily be achieved by providing a specific children's corner, which needs only to contain one or two small chairs and a table on which are placed children's books or comics, building bricks, plasticine, puzzles and other activity toys. A small blackboard and chalk often provide a welcome diversion. Posters should not be dental but of subjects to which children can relate, such as cartoon or comic characters. All these facilities absorb the children's concentration and make visiting the dentist an occasion to look forward to—with a consequent positive effect on attendance figures.

If the waiting room is large enough, a custom-built children's corner can be provided with a work surface and small chairs, of a suitable height for children, built into one side of the waiting room. This has the advantage of keeping the children's activities separate from the main adult waiting area. If space within the practice permits it, a complete children's play area can be provided. This could be more of an activity than a seated play area, and would clearly be extremely attractive to children, encourage them to visit the dentist, and give them a happier approach to dental treatment.

It is also helpful to provide a small pinboard on which photographs of young patients can be placed. 'A smile of the week' competition could be a feature, showing half a dozen pictures of smiling children, with the week's winner marked accordingly.

It is clear that provision of a children's corner or play area results in a more relaxed and cooperative patient; however, there is an additional advantage. Parents can see that the dentist has given thought to the children's welfare and it clearly demonstrates to them that he is a caring dentist. This often becomes a talking point among them and their friends and can result in new patients being attracted to the practice.

Uniforms

Every member of staff should be dressed neatly and

tidily and present the correct image of the practice to the patient. The choice of colour and design of uniforms is very much a personal one but, whatever is chosen, there should be a standard colour and design for every member of staff, including the dentist. Many now favour pastel colours for uniforms; others prefer white since it implies cleanliness and hygiene, which they feel is particularly important in these times of public concern about infection control. However, an all-white uniform can look cold and clinical and, if this is the uniform of choice, it should be relieved by the use of brightly coloured belts and trimmings.

The most practical uniform for the dentist and chairside staff is a coloured top with white trousers. This combines a bright, attractive look with the appearance of cleanliness and hygiene. Female chairside staff may prefer to wear a dress rather than trousers. This should be of a material which is the same colour and pattern as the top of the clinical uniform worn by the dentist. It is preferable for the reception staff to wear non-clinical outfits. These should be smart and business-like. With two or more receptionists working together, their outfits should match.

It has been said that one sends signals by the clothes one wears. The correct choice suggests success, the poor choice, mediocrity.

Staff uniforms convey the message of a 'team' approach to patient care. The uniform tells the patients that the individual is part of a group and this may help to restate source credibility in situations where ancillary staff are required to communicate information to patients.

It should be obvious that female members of staff should only wear very light make-up and have short unpolished nails and a neat and tidy hairstyle.

Conclusion

This can all perhaps be best summarized by paying attention to use of the senses to determine whether the image presented fulfils the correct criteria. There is but one chance to make a good first impression. A lasting impression is important, as the patient may well mention this to potential new patients.

On coming into the practice each day, the dentist might consider taking a general impression, as the patient will do on entering the building:

● Look—colour, size, shape and brightness.
● Touch—smoothness, softness.
● Smell—freshness, absence of 'clinical' odours.
● Listen—pitch and volume of sounds within the practice.

Careful attention to all the aspects of practice image discussed will undoubtedly prove to be an important factor in attracting and retaining patients. First, it will reassure the patients by looking familiar and as much like the patients' home surroundings as possible. Secondly, being a little different to other practices could well pay dividends, since the patients will talk to their friends and family about the practice and its decor. Finally, it will provide a pleasant, relaxed atmosphere for both the dentist and his staff, who should feel content to spend their working life in a pleasant environment of which they can be proud, with a consequent improvement in both morale and efficiency.

2 Marketing dentistry—the practice builder

Dentists in many countries are experiencing a fall in the demand for dental treatment. This is associated with a drop in practice gross income and consequently, as overheads are rising, with a decrease in practice profitability and the dentist's own disposable income. The solution can only be to increase the demand for dental treatment.

It must be recognized that the need for a great deal of treatment does exist. Unfortunately there is still a very large percentage of the population who visit the dentist either infrequently or not at all. Every practice needs to communicate effectively with both its regular and occasional patients. If it is to grow, it must endeavour to encourage positive attitudes and gain acceptance and approval of its services.

The aim of every dentist should be to increase the demand for dentistry within regular patients of the practice by ensuring through good internal marketing that *all* patients are aware of *all* services available. At the same time, he should aim to increase the overall number of patients by attracting the non- or infrequent attender. It must be emphasized that patients can only be educated if the dentist first establishes a rapport of trust with them and makes them receptive to information. The dentist must understand the needs of his patients and address himself to meeting those needs. For example, the increasing public interest in cosmetic dentistry presents an ideal service for the progressive dentist to market to existing patients.

Those prepared to invest time and money into their efforts and to market properly their dental practices are finding the public is willing to listen, and that patient demand, far from falling, is in most cases steadily increasing.

Marketing of dental services may be defined as the management process responsible for identifying, anticipating and satisfying patient needs profitably and ethically. There is nothing shameful about using the word 'marketing' in this context and it is not in conflict with professional dignity provided, of course, that it is honest. Marketing can be divided into external (mailing of practice brochures, press advertising, etc) and internal (making existing patients aware of techniques, materials and products available within the dentist's own practice).

It has to be clearly understood that marketing is not exactly the same as 'selling'. The latter is understandably something which many dentists are reluctant to do. Only through the application of successful marketing strategies can dentists hope to meet the competitive challenges facing them, improve their financial future and enhance their professional image. The primary objectives are:

- To determine the wants and needs of the target population.
- To make that population aware that the practice exists, through the appropriate means, or 'message'.
- To ensure that patients understand the message sent by the practice.
- To relate the message to their needs. Patients buy benefits, not features.
- To convince patients that the practice has honesty and integrity.
- To achieve patient satisfaction more effectively and efficiently than competitors (that is, other dentists).

Professional excellence is the only way to develop and expand the dental practice. Satisfaction of the target population gains loyalty from

Table 2.1 Problems and solutions in patient attendance.

Problems	Solutions
REGULAR PATIENTS	
- lack of patient awareness	- improving communication
- failure of dentist	- updating service
- financial constraints	- improving payment facilities
OCCASIONAL OR NON-ATTENDERS	
- fear	- patient reassurance
- lack of patient awareness	- improving communication
	- patient education
- financial constraints	- improving payment facilities
- time	- adapting practice hours

patients, continued patronage and favourable comments to non-patients.

In relation to the potential for dental treatment, the population may be broadly divided into three categories:

● Those who regularly attend for treatment.
● Those who occasionally attend—usually for relief of pain.
● Those who never attend.

There is an enormous amount of treatment potential existing in all three categories which is not being fully realized. Because all three have different attitudes and needs, that potential has to be realized in different ways. Therefore the reasons why all treatment needs are not being met should first be examined for each category and the appropriate solutions then applied (Table 2.1). The value of treatment planning and the nature of the market will be discussed later in the chapter (pages 21–4 and 24–6).

Improving communication

Lack of awareness by the patient of changing trends in dental care—particularly in the areas of preventive and cosmetic dentistry—is often the fault of the dentist because of poor communication with the patient. There is a failure to educate the patient positively in the different types of treatment which modern dentistry offers and to acquaint him with new materials and techniques. The patient may

attend regularly but the dentist contents himself with rendering only routine maintenance—often confined to basic restorative treatment.

The solution is accordingly to improve communication. Not only does this provide a positive education for the patient but it also stimulates the dentist to keep up with changing trends in dentistry. This is a significant factor with both regular and occasional patients. It is therefore important to discuss the various methods of achieving this in some detail.

Communication may be divided into:

● Verbal
● Written
● Visual (including audio-visual)

Verbal communication

This is the most basic though least effective method of education. Furthermore, some dentists may find difficulty in talking to patients and expressing themselves clearly. The purpose of talking to patients about their treatment is to increase their awareness of the parameters of modern dentistry. Few patients are aware of what is available in terms of modern materials and techniques, and it is to the advantage of every dentist and member of staff to remedy this omission.

It is essential to talk about the services, techniques and materials available, their differences, the procedures they involve, and the advantages and disadvantages of each. For example, in discussing posterior composite fillings, it is important not only to point out the cosmetic difference but to emphasize the important advantage of actually bonding the material to the tooth structure. Often this is much more of a motivating factor for patient acceptance than the solely cosmetic advantage.

Consultation area

Patient education and motivation should take place away from the immediate clinical treatment area. The decisive factor in accepting or rejecting treatment is not what the dentist says, but what the patient hears and understands. Bearing in mind the degree of apprehension of the average dental patient, any attempt at verbal communication will be affected if the patient is spoken to while seated in the dental chair. The fact that the patient is in the place that he fears most will almost certainly ensure that the greater proportion of the information given by the dentist is not absorbed. For this reason, all verbal communication should take place in an area entirely separate from the immediate chairside. Such an area is referred to as a consultation area.

If possible, the consultation area should be a totally separate room but, if space precludes this, a section of the treatment area itself can be demarcated for the purpose. Whether the area is a separate room or a section of the treatment area itself, certain basic principles must be observed:

- It should be decorated in a different yet bright and relaxing style, and look totally non-dental (see Chapter 1).
- It should contain a desk and chairs. The chairs should preferably be arranged so that dentist and patient can sit side by side. If the chairs are placed on either side of the desk, the patient may feel dominated.
- The chairs should ensure that dentist and patient sit at the same height.
- The desk should have an X-ray viewer and a daylight viewer for slides. All study and demonstration models should be readily accessible.

A large-size, back-projection film viewer is particularly valuable. Not only is it very useful for the diagnosis of X-ray films but it may be used to show to the patient both slides of treated cases, which relate to the particular treatment he is to have and the patient's own X-ray films. Showing a patient his own X-ray photographs on a large screen, with, for example, hidden interproximal cavities or loss of crestal bone, can be an extremely valuable aid to patient motivation.

One other important point must be emphasized. Not only must patient education be given an area separate from the dental chair but a specific time must be set aside for it. Most attempts at patient education made during treatment procedures will fail because patients do not absorb information if they are not relaxed. The problem is that because talking does not produce a specific end-result in terms of an item of treatment, and therefore a fee,

the dentist feels such time is wasted. This is a totally erroneous view because time spent in talking to patients can often be extremely productive in terms of future treatment.

Written communication

It is generally accepted that written information is more effectively retained than that given verbally. All verbal patient education must therefore be reinforced with written aids of various types. These may consist of:

- Practice brochure
- Practice stationery
- Educational pamphlets and brochures
- Posters
- Books

Practice brochure

Every dental practice must now provide a brochure. This is one of the most valuable and easiest methods of patient motivation and education. A well-produced brochure not only tells both existing and prospective patients about the type of treatment and facilities available but it also helps to convey the distinctive practice image, which will attract new patients. It is an excellent yet simple way of providing an introduction to modern dental techniques and of promoting the practice and its services. A wide range of commercially produced brochures are available which are personalized by overprinting the dentist's own name and address. Alternatively, the dentist can design and print his own brochure. It is helpful to do this in conjunction with senior practice staff and a good designer. The style of the contents should be friendly, easily read and understood, and not over-long. All brochures should be updated at least annually and should include new techniques and facilities offered by the practice.

The practice brochure should include the following basic facts:

- Name of the principal dentist, permanent partners and hygienist. The names of other associates and staff members should not feature since such staff members may leave and so make the brochure outdated.

- Address and telephone number of the practice.
- Hours of opening. These should be particularly emphasized if they extend beyond normal office hours, and if the practice is open at weekends.
- Emergency phone numbers which will provide a 24-hour cover.
- Details of the recall system used in the practice.
- Details of how charges are based and arrangements for payment of fees.
- Types and names of insurance schemes for which cover is provided.

Motivational statements of the following type should be included:

- Welcome to the practice. A statement of practice policy should be given.
- The most modern types of equipment and materials are used.
- Techniques used in the practice are at the forefront of dental technology. (A brief description should be given of some of the newer techniques which are available in the practice, for example adhesive bridges, porcelain veneering and light-cured cosmetic restorations.)
- Patients requiring emergency treatment are guaranteed to be treated on the same day as they call.
- The practice welcomes children.
- Preventive dentistry is high on the list of priorities for the practice.
- Sedation techniques are available where required.
- Domiciliary visits are made.
- The practice takes strict precautions against cross-infection. (Mention must be made of the use of disposable needles and materials, autoclaving and the wearing of gloves.)

Every patient of the practice must receive the practice brochure. The most effective way is to mail the brochures out, either individually or included with recalls and accounts. Alternatively the dentist may give one to each patient personally at the recall examination. New patients should be mailed a practice brochure immediately after they have telephoned for an appointment. This ensures that they are familiar with the basic principles and method of organization of the practice before they arrive for the initial appointment.

Practice brochures can also be sent out unsolicited as a random mail-shot, where local regulations allow this. A local mailing firm could be employed to mail out the practice brochure to non-patients in the immediate catchment area of the practice. This is more cost-effective in terms of patient return than advertising in newspapers or magazines. Furthermore, if the practice brochure is mailed to existing patients, it may also be seen by other members of the family and/or friends who may not currently be patients of the practice. Done with taste, this can increase public awareness and produce new patients. Like their colleagues in other professions, dentists are now finding that costly advertising in national newspapers, magazines and telephone directories is relatively ineffective in attracting significant numbers of patients. Such advertising is better confined to school, parent-teacher association and parish magazines and local newspapers. While these have low circulations, they attract a high level of attention, are inexpensive and are likely to be far more productive in attracting patients.

In addition to a brochure, some dentists publish a regular newsletter. This can be printed, or typed and photocopied. The newsletter could include news about members of staff (such as new additions, marriages, babies) and information about new facilities, materials and techniques being used in the practice. There should be a short section for children, which might include such features as puzzles and competitions. A newsletter provides an excellent public relations service and helps to project the image of a caring, family practice as well as being a very positive vehicle for patient education.

Practice stationery

Visiting cards, notepaper, appointment cards and reminder cards should be carefully designed and printed to present an attractive modern image. The dentist might consider the use of a visual symbol or logo to represent the image of the practice and the services it offers. Apart from being decorative, a carefully designed logo gives an individual identity to the practice and also conveys a message which is easily understood by patients. This logo should then be reproduced on every item of practice notepaper, brochures, business and reminder cards, appointment cards and invoices. It helps to make the practice distinctive and attractive.

Some thought might also be given to lending the practice a 'corporate' identity. Rather than having the name of the dentist or dentists on stationery, it might be better to give the practice a title which could be based on the name of the building, road, or area in which it is situated. For example, 'John Doe Dentist' projects the image of a small, single-handed practice, while 'Columbus Square Dental Practice' might well convey to a patient the image of a larger practice, with a larger range of facilities.

The appointment card itself merits special attention because it must project a good image of the practice and be regarded as another form of low-key advertising. Thus care should be taken in its design and content. An alternative to the conventional single-sided card is one of a large size, folded over to produce four pages. The front has the practice details and logo, the back has spaces for appointments and the card opens to show two pages of practice information (Figure 2.1). This should include the important statements that:

- High priority is given to preventive dentistry.
- Children are treated. (Patients are often under the mistaken impression that many dentists do not like to treat children.)
- Dentistry can be painless.

Figure 2.1

The information printed on the inside of the appointment card introduces the practice and its policy. The message is one which is likely to encourage patients to attend.

WELCOME to our practice, where we hope to offer you total dental care in a relaxed and friendly atmosphere.

CHILDREN are most welcome and are never too young to have their first visit.

PREVENTION is our aim. We would like to see all children growing up with perfect teeth in a healthy mouth.

COSMETICS are important. There are modern techniques of bonding which can dramatically improve your dental appearance. Please do not hesitate to consult us, no matter how trivial the problem may seem to you. Many of these techniques do not involve removal of tooth material, so no injection or drilling is required.

STERILIZATION. Wherever possible, new disposable items are used for each patient. All other instruments are sterilized by autoclaving. All dentists and assistants wear gloves when working on patients.

FINALLY, we realized that you may be worried about visiting the dentist for a variety of reasons. If there is anything that worries you, about any aspect of treatment, please do not hesitate to talk to us about it.

- Modern techniques are used.
- The dentist and staff are sympathetic to the fears of potential patients and take great care in helping to allay those fears.

Another advantage of this type of appointment card is that its size and design makes it less likely to be mislaid or lost, so reducing the potential for failed appointments. Other possibilities to be considered in appointment card design are to print it in an attractive colour, and include a simple map showing directions to the practice, bus and train routes and car-parking facilities.

Educational pamphlets and brochures

There are a wide range of pre-printed brochures produced commercially that explain in easy-to-understand language the various aspects of dental treatment available today. Among those readily available are the series produced by the American Dental Association, the British Dental Health Foundation and many commercial companies. These can usually be overprinted with the dentist's own name and address, so making them more personal. They should be mailed out to patients with recalls and accounts, and supplies left both at reception and in the waiting area for patients to take away. These brochures often stimulate patients to request details of various types of treatment before the dentist or staff have even discussed it with them. Such brochures are not intended to be the sole method of patient education but are certainly of value as an introduction. The danger of over-saturating the patient with information must be avoided by keeping the number of topics covered to a minimum. All pamphlets and brochures must be neatly placed in an attractive rack, located in an eye-catching position.

As an alternative to brochures, it is now possible to obtain laminated 'trigger' cards containing information about every procedure undertaken in a dental office, written in layman's language and including simple colour illustrations. Placed in custom-made wall racks, trigger cards can be very eye-catching. They also have the advantage of being relatively permanent, since their laminated surface does not become worn. The disadvantage is that they can only be read in the waiting room and cannot be taken home, so that the patient's friends and family do not see the material.

Posters

It is a matter of some debate whether wall posters in the waiting area have a place as a method of patient education. In general, patients absorb very little information from posters. Moreover posters have the disadvantage of making the waiting area look too clinical and detract from the relaxing atmosphere, which is so important. It is perhaps better to limit this type of information to a small noticeboard which can carry a variety of objects, such as small pamphlets, 'before' and 'after' photographs of cases treated by the dentist, patient information, favourable magazine articles dealing with dentistry, letters of appreciation from patients and any interesting news items about the dentist or staff.

Books

Of particular value in the waiting room is a *patient information book*, or ring-binder, which can be made up by the dentist himself. The first few pages should have photographs and very brief biographical details about the dentist and every member of the staff. Subsequent pages would contain 'before' and 'after' photographs of actual cases treated in the practice, with a very simple description of the treatment. This information is of great value in promoting the patients' knowledge of available techniques and particularly in showing the results of cosmetic procedures (see also page 17).

Commercially produced books, for example *Change your smile* (Goldstein, 1988) and *Smile portfolio* (Ibsen, 1986), deal mainly with cosmetic dentistry and have the distinct advantage of showing cases by presenting full-face photographs. It is found that patients identify much more readily with this method of illustration than with intra-oral close-up views of the mouth. This should also be borne in mind when the dentist is preparing his own book.

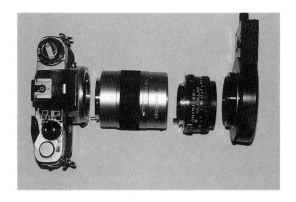

Figure 2.2

The single-lens reflex camera showing the body, macro-converter, lens and ringflash.

Visual communication

Photographs

Photographs are a simple and effective form of communication, both inside and outside the treatment area. A Polaroid CU-5 dental close-up camera is particularly useful for the dentist who is not an accomplished photographer. This is simple to use, being purely automatic and, in most practices, the dental assistant (DA) can take both the pre- and post-operative photograph.

As an alternative, a conventional camera can be converted into a clinical photography kit and is cheaper than the Polaroid system. The kit comprises a 35 mm single-lens reflex camera body and lens, macro-converter and ringflash (Figure 2.2). The system is extremely easy to use and by simply changing the setting on the converter, high-quality colour prints or slides can be produced, which range from a full-face view to a close-up of only six anterior teeth.

The advantages of photography are as follows:

- It makes the patient aware of the need for treatment by emphasizing dental defects. Discolouration, rotation, recession, staining and irregularities may all be dramatically demonstrated to the patient. With Polaroid photography, an immediate result may be obtained within 60 seconds of taking the photograph. The need for treatment is thereby demonstrated immediately.

- If a new patient's first visit is with the dentist, two instant Polaroid prints should be made by the DA. One is kept with the patient's records and the other is given to the patient to take home. It has been noted that this photograph is shown to spouses and friends. The result is often a call from the patient asking if they can bring in a husband, wife or friend for consultation (Altshuler, 1989). This is an excellent example of subliminal marketing.

- Where the initial visit is with the hygienist, photographs may be taken at that time and used to bring to the patient's attention any defects which may present. The hygienist may then suggest discussing the possibility of improvement with the dentist at the next appointment. In this way, it is easier for the dentist to motivate the patient, as the latter has been made aware that an improvement can be effected.

- Such photographs can be used as an efficient marketing tool for explaining principles, procedures and examples of the types of treatment available. (Altshuler, Johnson, Manzoli, 1983).

- Photographs of the completed treatment can be shown with the pre-operative one and used in the patient information book displayed in the waiting area. People relate more to photographs that they know to be of fellow patients of the same practice than they do to those in the commercially produced brochures. The credibility of the dentist is enhanced by pictures of work which he himself has done. Patients are more likely to be reassured of the dentist's capability by seeing his own work rather than that of an anonymous operator.

The need for good dental photography is becoming increasingly important in general practice, particularly in the area of patient motivation.

A detailed consideration of the subject is outside the scope of this book and the reader is referred to one of the excellent books now available (for example, Wander and Gordon, 1988).

Videos

Videos are becoming a valuable means of patient education. Their main advantages are:

● Visual communication is many times faster than written or verbal, and the information contained is absorbed more effectively and remembered for far longer.
● When shown in the waiting area, videos save valuable dentist and staff time.
● Patients accept the video presentation as an impartial third party.
● Staff can show and explain procedures while watching the video with the patient. Patients tend to relate to staff far more than to the dentist and ask them for guidance and opinions about treatment. This often leaves the dentist with little more to say in order to gain patient acceptance of the procedure.
● Treatment procedures are clearly demonstrated and all the positive advantages of a particular treatment are emphasized.
● Knowledge of the procedure is provided in the best possible light and allows the patient to arrive at a balanced decision.
● Patients often relate to the actors featured in the video.
● Children in particular identify with a TV screen and this is especially effective in getting across the message of preventive dentistry and diet control.

A wide range of patient education videotapes are now available commercially. These should be used in two ways:

● Kept constantly running in the waiting room. The principal advantage of this is that it stimulates initial awareness and interest in modern techniques and encourages patients to discuss them with the dentist.
● Shown in the consultation area by the dentist or staff member to explain a specific treatment directly to an individual patient. Videotapes can be used to motivate, to help clarify precisely what a procedure entails, or to reinforce previous verbal explanation.

Models

Three-dimensional models are even more effective than photographs or leaflets. Perhaps the simplest and yet most valuable models are those using casts of the patient's own mouth. Misplaced, rotated, tilted or over-erupted teeth show up much more dramatically on such models and can be seen far better by the patient than the actual teeth, viewed in a mirror. For example a model showing a patient's molar over-erupted into an opposing space is much more likely to motivate him to accept posterior bridgework than merely showing him the space in his own mouth—particularly if this is not of great cosmetic concern to him.

Another simple model can be made by the dentist or his assistant by mounting four extracted molar teeth in a block of acrylic, leaving one untreated but with deep fissures, and restoring one with a fissure sealant, one with amalgam and one with a posterior composite filling (Figure 2.3). Such a model is effective because treated and untreated teeth are shown together to the patient. By allowing the patient to see and handle such a model, the difference between a deep, untreated fissure and one which has been fissure sealed, for example, will be strikingly obvious. This will be of far greater significance, and therefore more likely to be accepted, than a verbal description. Few parents would then fail to accept the cost of fissure sealing for their childrens' teeth.

More sophisticated models can be made by the dental technician or obtained commercially (Figure 2.4). Such models show clearly the various types of crowns, bridges (both fixed and adhesive), porcelain veneers and gold, porcelain or composite inlays. Models can also be obtained commercially showing, for example, the various degrees of periodontal disease, malocclusions, and deciduous and adult dentitions.

Updating service

The dentist may fail to see changing needs and to keep abreast of new trends in dental care. The

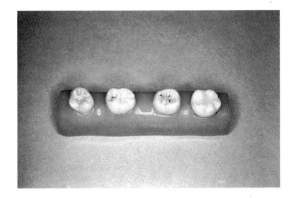

Figure 2.3

Four extracted molar teeth mounted in acrylic showing one untreated, one fissure sealed, one restored with an amalgam filling.

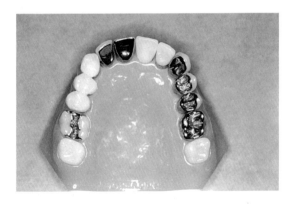

Figure 2.4

A commercially produced demonstration model showing an inlay and various types of crowns and bridgework.

current trend, for example, is to emphasize cosmetic and preventive dentistry rather than restorative. The dentist fails to see alternative areas of treatment which the patient may want if only he knew about them. Patients will not ask for treatment of which they are unaware.

The practice base must be broadened to offer a wider range of techniques, services and facilities to existing patients. For this reason, the dentist must constantly update his knowledge and skills to ensure that he is able to offer all the most modern techniques. The patient in turn will often act as a missionary and refer in other new patients.

Improving payment facilities

Patients may be unwilling or genuinely unable to find the capital necessary for the treatment. This is compounded by the failure of many patients to place dental treatment high on their list of priorities. Ways of spreading the cost must be provided by offering facilities for settlement by such means as credit cards, standing orders, insurance schemes and deferred payments. This is discussed more fully in Chapter 4.

Patients who are infrequent attenders often have a totally erroneous idea of the cost of dental treatment. The overall impression is that it is usually very expensive. Every patient must be clearly informed at the beginning of treatment of the total cost which will be involved. Treatment must never be commenced without the patient having an absolutely clear idea of the expenditure and method of payment accepted by the practice. This is dealt with in more detail in Chapter 4. By giving patients the opportunity of spreading payments over a period, treatment is often accepted which would otherwise be rejected because of the difficulty of finding immediate capital.

As an example, a colleague decided one of his patients had an 'attitude problem' because she was in two minds whether to pay the fee quoted for a course of treatment. The dentist thought that the fee discussed was a bargain and could not understand why she would not accept his proposal. He failed to realize that the attitude problem was his and not the patient's. The fee represented one month's disposable income for that particular patient. The same patient visited another practice where the dentist made a similar recommendation but understood the dilemma. He allowed her credit facilities to spread payment over a number of months and the patient accepted the whole course of treatment.

Patient reassurance

Fear of pain is the all too common reason underlying irregular attendance. Perhaps the most basic solution is to remove the fear of dentists and convey the message that modern dentistry can be virtually painless. For this reason, it is particularly important to treat children with great care and to avoid physical trauma totally. A clean, modern practice and a warm, friendly staff often displace negative childhood memories of the dentist. The importance of providing an environment in which all patients can feel relaxed has been fully discussed in Chapter 1.

When new patients attend for the first time, and before seating them in the dental chair, it is vital that the dentist should talk to them for a few minutes in the consultation room or area. A few minutes spent discussing their reasons for attending, likes and dislikes, fear and immediate problems, as well as a little of their personal background, will do wonders to relax the patients and make them much more at ease before treatment commences.

If time permits, it is important to complete a simple but painless procedure on the new patient's first visit. Wherever possible, this should be a non-invasive and cosmetic procedure, such as the restoration of a cervical erosion area. In the absence of such lesions, an alternative is to restore a small occlusal cavity in an upper premolar. This can be of enormous value in building confidence and removing fear. The use of surface anaesthetic and a local injection with a thin, 30 g needle makes both the anaesthesia and the filling totally painless.

It is also accepted that patients are less apprehensive and more conducive to accepting dental treatment if the dentist carefully explains what the treatment will involve and also talks to them during treatment and tells them what he is doing.

Patient education

There is an unfortunate tendency in large numbers of the population to accept poor dental health (including cavities, periodontal disease and poor cosmetics) as a normal fact of life. These patients tend only to visit the dentist when in pain. This attitude is by no means isolated to the lower socio-economic class of the population. The problem is compounded by the many false ideas which seem to have developed among the public, for example: 'fillings fall out'; 'dentistry is painful'; 'denture clasps cause decay in teeth'.

It must be accepted that prejudices and misconceptions about dental treatment can really only be removed through a concerted nationwide education programme. However, individual dentists can help by taking the time to talk to patients who attend their practice for casual treatment. A sympathetic manner coupled with the removal of acute pain often converts a casual to a regular patient. This can also be supplemented by giving talks to Rotary Clubs, schools, youth and other communal organizations and by writing articles for both the local and national press.

Adapting practice hours

The patient may genuinely want to attend regularly but finds it difficult to do so during working hours because either he is not allowed to take time off or, if he does so, he will lose his pay for that time.

Dentists must now appreciate the need to work 'people' hours by providing early morning, late evening or even weekend appointments. Such hours are found to be extremely popular and so act as a very valuable practice builder by catering for those people who would otherwise be unable to attend.

In addition, practice hours can be staggered. For example, on one or two days, the dentist may prefer to be free in the morning and work from 2.00 pm to 9.00 pm. Where there are several partners or associates, the practice could be worked on a two session per day basis, that is, with one dentist working from 8.00 am until 2.00 pm and the second working from 2.00 pm until 8.00 pm. This makes maximum use of the facilities.

It is certainly preferable to allowing expensive equipment to stand idle for a long proportion of the day.

Treatment planning

The importance of countering lack of patient awareness and failure to appreciate the need for treatment has been emphasized. Treatment planning is essential to ensure that the patient is made fully aware of all the treatment required for full dental fitness and so realize his full treatment potential. It also acts as a very effective vehicle for dental education. Treatment planning should always be applied to every new patient and to certain categories of existing patients. There are four distinct stages involved:

● Pre-clinical and clinical examinations
● Case study
● Consultation
● Written confirmation

Stage 1: preclinical and clinical examinations

The first meeting with a new patient should always be in the consultation area. Assuming that both the record card and the medical history form have been completed, a number of specific questions must be asked and the answers noted briefly on the record card. These might comprise:

● The patient's immediate reason for attending.
● Previous dental history. This will often elicit details of any unpleasant experiences, fears or phobias. This is particularly important so that the dentist can take care to avoid repetition.
● Any particular aspects of dentistry disliked by the patient.
● The patient's occupation.
● Any potential problems or difficulties relating to appointment times or days.
● The name of the person recommending or referring the patient. This person should subsequently be thanked with a personal letter from the dentist.
● Any interesting personal information, such as a proposed trip abroad, a son or daughter taking

exams, a new job. A follow-up question on that information at a subsequent visit implies personal identification with the patient and converts them from a file number to a person. In the same way, who can fail to be impressed at being greeted by name by the *Maître d'* of a large restaurant? However, he has probably glanced at his reservation book just a few seconds before.

At this point, a form can be given to the patient which has questions on the patient's own feelings about his or her smile and the general appearance of his or her teeth. Such forms are available commercially. This is completed by the patient personally and can reveal very valuable information. It may even help to heighten the patient's awareness of conditions which had hitherto seemed either insignificant or untreatable. At the very least, it helps to promote the image of the dentist as a caring professional. Many dentists prefer the patient to complete this particular form at the same time as the medical history form. This means that both forms are available to the dentist before the patient enters the consultation area.

This preclinical examination may only take a few minutes but establishes an initial rapport between the dentist and patient and clearly projects the image of a caring dentist. This helps the patient to be more relaxed for the next step—the clinical examination.

A full clinical examination follows, including identification of caries incidence, plaque score, periodontal condition and pocket depth, and full-mouth intra-oral and panoral X-ray photographs are taken. The patient should then be given a large mirror and actually shown any visible cavities, spaces due to missing teeth, staining, irregularities, plaque, bleeding and calculus. Defective contact points should be demonstrated by the dentist using floss on the patient's own teeth while he looks in the mirror. Patients often consider irregularities of teeth, bleeding, spaces and defective contacts a normal fact of life which therefore do not need to be treated. However, it must be emphasized that once the dentist can demonstrate to the patient that such conditions are not normal, that treatment is required, and that the dentist can provide it, the patient will almost invariably accept this. Other than pain, fear of losing teeth is after all a major factor in motivating patients to seek treatment. If at this stage an obvious need is apparent for more complex treatment, such as crowns, bridges, veneers, orthodontics or prosthetics, impression for study models should be taken, preferably with a face-bow registration for mounting on an anatomical articulator.

Regular patients should undergo a routine recall examination. If it becomes apparent that more complex treatment is required, for example to improve cosmetic appearance, to insert bridgework following tooth loss or to deal with teeth or restorations badly fractured since the last recall visit, the treatment plan should be used in precisely the same way with the exception that the preclinical examination is omitted.

Stage 2: Case study

The dentist must study the patient's charts, mounted study casts and X-ray films and plan the different courses of treatment of varying complexity which are available to treat the particular case. He should never prejudge the patient's ability to pay when planning the treatment.

All the alternatives must be carefully noted and each one costed by the dentist on the basis of the practice fee system. They should range from the most complex to the most simple solution to the particular problem. For example, when restoring edentulous spaces, it may be that the same patient could be treated by either fixed bridgework, precision-attached removable bridgework, cast-metal removable dentures or adhesive bridgework. Each would therefore be listed with the fee appropriate to it.

Mounted models are very important diagnostic aids, helping the dentist to observe any potential problems such as over-erupted or tilted teeth, plunger cusps, or unfavourable occlusion which may not have been apparent on clinical examination. If porcelain veneers are to be considered, such models can facilitate decisions on the feasibility, amount and sites of any enamel reduction required, and difficult paths of insertion due to undercuts, which can easily be corrected by marking these sites on the model itself. The models may also be used for cases requiring bridgework to wax up pontics or irregular teeth for veneers so that the potential for correction is more easily observed.

Finally, should the patient elect to have fixed crown or bridgework, the models may be used for the laboratory construction of temporary shells.

Stage 3: Consultation

Some days after the initial examination, the patient should attend for a consultation appointment. The patient's partner or parent may also wish to be present, particularly if he or she is the financial provider. The appointment should take place in the consultation area.

The dentist should discuss all the alternatives in the treatment plan evolved in Stage 2. Each alternative must be carefully explained with the factors for and against it, and the different fees carefully presented. At this stage, the use of visual aids is particularly important. If treatment is likely to be complex, prolonged and costly, it is often helpful to divide the total plan into phases. Phase 1 would be treatment needed to be completed urgently, such as caries, scaling and periodontal therapy, endodontics or occlusal adjustment. Subsequent phases of treatment would be listed in descending order of priority. This helps to spread the total cost over a period of time and, if such a facility is offered to the patient, it may sometimes make the difference between acceptance and rejection of a treatment plan.

As phase 1 is often the least costly, some dentists prefer to discuss only this at the first consultation. The need for further dental treatment at a later date must, however, be referred to, albeit in fairly general terms. Discussion of these later phases can then be deferred until completion of phase 1, by which time the dentist will have established more of a rapport with the patient because treatment has commenced. Another advantage is that the patient is not presented with a possibly bewildering list of items of complex treatment. However, the patient must be aware at the outset that further treatment will be required in the future. The plan for this would be presented at a second consultation at a later date.

Should the patient accept one or other of the alternatives at the time of the consultation, an appropriate appointment may then be made. However, the patient may wish to give further thought and consideration to the treatment plan.

Dear [Patient Name]

TREATMENT PLAN

Following our discussion of [date], I write to confirm the treatment plan that we finalized. This will be as follows:-

Phase 1

Two visits to the Hygienist	(30 mins each)
Extraction of lower left first molar root	(30 mins)
Provisional bridge from lower left second premolar to second molar	(1 hour)
White fillings in upper right lateral incisor and canine	(1 hour)
Amalgam filling in upper left first molar	(30 mins)

Five visits will be required.

Fee for Phase 1: [X]

Phase 2 (six months after completion of phase 1)

One visit to the Hygienist
Prepare permanent bridge in porcelain bonded to gold from lower left second premolar to second molar   (1 hour)
Fit bridge

Three visits required.

Fee for Phase 2: [Y]

In accordance with our practice custom, 50 per cent of the fee is payable at the first visit and the balance on completion of each phase.

If there is anything further that you wish me to clarify, please do not hesitate to contact me.

We look forward to seeing you for your first appointment at [time] on [date] when [Name], our Hygienist, will begin your scaling and gum treatment.

With kind regards.

Sincerely yours

[Dentist Name]

Figure 2.5

An individually typed confirmation letter of a treatment plan accepted by verbal agreement. This contains full details of proposed treatment including duration and number of appointments required. The fees and method of payment are clearly stated.

In this case, the final decision can be given by the patient over the telephone or, if necessary, at a further short consultation appointment.

The payment policy of the practice must be clearly discussed at this consultation appointment and the method of payment by the patient clearly established at this time.

Stage 4: Written confirmation

When a final decision has been made, details of the plan chosen must be put in writing and sent to the

Dear

Further to our recent consultation, I have pleasure in quoting the fee of .... for the following treatment:

I trust that this will be acceptable and I shall be pleased to receive your confirmation in due course. If there are any points requiring clarification, please do not hesitate to contact me.

Yours sincerely

Figure 2.6

A pre-printed confirmation letter. The details of treatment and fees would be typed in for each patient.

patient with a copy kept by the dentist in the patient's records. The confirmation letter would comprise:

- Brief description of the proposed treatment divided into phases and stages.
- Sequence of treatment to be followed.
- Number of appointments.
- Treatment to be delivered at each.
- Time required for each appointment.
- If the treatment is divided into phases, the interval between each.
- Total fee and agreed method of payment.
- Statement that some modification to the original plan may be needed as treatment progresses.

The copy of plan which is mailed to the patient could be bound, for example in a clear plastic cover

with a slide-on plastic spine. This shows the patient clearly that care, time and attention have been put into its preparation.

Figure 2.5 shows a typical confirmation letter. It will be noted that the emphasis is on the method of payment, as well as the amount. In particular, the phrase 'in accordance with our practice custom' makes it clear to the patient that this is the standard procedure adopted for all patients and he is not being singled out as untrustworthy or a credit risk!

By using a word processor, a standard letter may be formulated that can be adapted to incorporate the individual details for each patient. The alternative is a preprinted letter in which only the treatment details and the cost are inserted (Figure 2.6). This is a great deal less personal and does not contain the detail of the individualized letter.

Written confirmation is mandatory in order to prevent the possibility of misunderstandings, which are all too frequent if verbal communication is used alone. Moreover fees tend to be much more acceptable to patients when a well-organized treatment plan is presented in an understandable way.

It may at first appear that this four-stage treatment plan is unduly complex and time-consuming. If properly organized, it does not in fact need to be so, and it should in any event be regarded as an important means of promoting public relations, patient education and motivation. It is extremely effective in motivating patients to accept treatment which they would not otherwise have accepted. The time spent is thus potentially very productive.

Market segmentation

The available market is not a single entity but made up of different social and economic groups, which are therefore segments of the whole. This concept of market segmentation is the key to successful marketing of the dental practice. The different groups must be approached in different ways to avoid any waste of time and costs, and to maximize the effectiveness for each individual group.

Children

Positive practice promotions must be used. These will vary slightly according to the age group.

Every practice must have an area for dental health education. One section should be fitted with sinks and large mirrors at which the hygienist or dental health educator can give supervised oral hygiene instructions and practice. It should be decorated in a style to which young children can relate and feel relaxed. For the same reason, the lighting should be warm and relaxing. Another section should be devoted to displays of incorrect and correct items of diet in relation to their cariogenic effect. This area should be used to show not only children but their parents the importance of correct diet in controlling caries.

A dental health club should be started. Membership cards and newsletters can be printed by the practice or alternatively the dentist can subscribe to one of the commercially organized clubs.

Children respond to positive encouragement, particularly when there is a tangible end-result. For example an appointment card can carry an incentive. A healthy mouth at the inspection appointment could gain a silver star, and three silver stars could entitle the child to a gold star and a badge, certificate or small gift. The prospect of a visible reward is a great incentive for children and usually ensures they maintain regular visits. Birthday cards may be sent to all child patients. Not only does this delight the child, but it is also good public relations. Cards can be obtained and then over-printed with the dentist's name and address. This advertises the practice to all the family and to the friends who visit the patient's house. Similarly, overprinted give-away presents such as crayons, colouring books, balloons and badges are greatly prized by children and are excellent publicity for the practice.

This type of scheme may be supplemented by using reminder cards specially directed at children obtainable from specialized dental stationery suppliers. These reminders must be addressed personally to the child, not the parent. Children receive little, if any, personal mail and the receipt of a communication personally addressed to them is not only more likely to ensure their attendance for the recall examination but also establishes a very personal rapport with the dentist. Studies have shown that personalized reminder cards increase the return of child patients (Woolgrove, Cumberbatch, Gelbier, 1988).

Another very productive promotional aid is to organize a number of 'children only' days within the practice. These should coincide with school holidays and on these days the practice should be open only to children. A letter to parents advising them of the event will ensure a good response. The success of such a day is assured by attention to a number of simple, temporary changes to the practice—for example:

- Change the pictures on the walls so that they appeal to children.
- Ensure children's magazines and toys are available.
- Eliminate clinical images such as white coats.
- Introduce repeating audio-visual materials and dental health education videos—these can be either serious or, more ideally, in cartoon form.
- Give out balloons, badges and stickers which can be overprinted with the dentist's name, address and/or a slogan.
- Give children the opportunity of watching other children receiving check-ups, advice and oral hygiene instruction. No operative procedures should be done at this visit. It has the advantage of showing clearly to children that dentistry can indeed be pleasant and pain-free.

Young children

A crèche can be provided so that young children can be brought and left while the parent has treatment. Either a member of the staff or a specific child-minder should be put in charge of this facility. Space for prams and pushchairs must be made available. Knowledge that such facilities are provided often serves to attract parents of young children to the practice.

Elderly people

Elderly patients have special needs which must be attended to in order to attract them to the practice. To this end, the caring dentist must ensure that:

- Access is good.
- On-site parking is available.
- Waiting room seating is comfortable but not too low (because of the effort required to rise from low seats).
- Domiciliary visits are available to those unable to leave their home.
- Appointment cards are designed with large, bold print for easy reading.

Ethnic groups

Any language barrier may cause a problem. If the practice is in or near a large ethnic community, consideration should be given to printing literature such as appointment cards, reminders, accounts and patient information in the mother tongue of that community. A member of staff should be engaged who speaks the ethnic mother tongue. This solves the problem of communicating explanations and instructions, some of which—oral hygiene instructions, for example—may be particularly hard to convey to a non-English speaker. Once it becomes known that such a person works within the practice, large numbers of the ethnic community will be attracted into seeking treatment.

Within the practice

As the need to stimulate demand must affect communication between practice and patient, it will also influence every aspect of management within the practice itself, from appearance through to communication between members of the team.

Environment

The importance of correct decor and design of the whole dental practice environment has been fully discussed in Chapter 1. Its value in practice building is that it gives the correct image of the dentist as an informed, caring dental practitioner and implies that every modern technique and material in dentistry is available to patients. For example, the offer of cosmetic dentistry is unlikely to gain acceptance with a patient in an environment which is not itself aesthetically pleasing.

Dentist and staff

It cannot be emphasized enough that every member of staff must at all times look smart, tidy and efficient and present a cheerful and warm demeanour to every patient. 'Service to our patients' should be the goal common to every member of staff (Table 2.7). It must never be forgotten that every patient, however long they have been with the practice, is to some degree a frightened and apprehensive individual. This is particularly important with new patients, especially if they are attending the practice for the relief of acute pain. Such patients can be converted from casual, infrequent attenders into regular patients by being exposed to a very relaxed and warm practice atmosphere and a caring, sympathetic and cheerful staff, and through the provision of treatment without discomfort or pain by the dentist.

Staff–patient relationship

- Every patient must be greeted with a smile and a pleasant voice.
- Communications between staff and patients must be purely by personal contact. Patients should be conducted to and from the treatment or consultation room by the member of staff responsible and never merely summoned over a telephone or intercom. This is far too impersonal.
- If the dentist is running late, the personal touch can be extended to taking a few minutes to go into the waiting room and letting the patient know. A reason should be given—patients do understand that procedures can become difficult. Supplementing this explanation with the offer of a hot drink further improves the relationship and can often defuse an awkward situation.

Figure 2.7 Memo to all practice personnel.

A PATIENT is the most important person in this practice, whether present in person, by correspondence or on the telephone.
The PATIENT is not dependent on us. We are dependent on him/her.
The PATIENT is not a statistic nor a mouth. He/she is a human being with feelings and emotions like our own.
The enquiring PATIENT is not an interruption of our work. He/she is the purpose of it.
We are not doing the PATIENT a favour by treating him/her. He/she is doing us a favour by giving us the opportunity to do so.

After Gordon Selfridge (founder of the famous London department store) in a memo to his staff.

- Every staff member must have a working knowledge of the different techniques, materials and services offered by the practice. Patients often question staff members about dentistry in preference to asking the dentist himself. This is usually because they are more relaxed with staff than with the dentist and find it easier to relate to them. This is particularly the case with reception staff, probably because they have the additional advantage that patients meet them in a totally non-clinical environment. It follows therefore that every member of staff, including receptionists, must be able to talk to patients about all the types of treatment available. It is mainly for this reason that staff must be taught about treatment, albeit at a relatively basic level. To this end, it is helpful for staff to attend relevant courses with the dentist. Apart from their educational value, they are useful as a means to motivate staff and to help enhance their self-esteem.
- The first contact a new patient has with the practice is usually over the telephone. A sympathetic telephone voice and a welcoming and courteous manner is a good ambassador for the dentist and can do much to create the right impression. This is dealt with in more detail in Chapter 3.

- Patients in pain must be seen as quickly as possible as a moral duty of the dentist. Moreover today's emergency patient may well be the permanent patient of the future. The initial visit of many patients to a dentist is prompted by acute pain. It is possible to separate out the genuine emergency by asking how long the patient has had the pain, whether it has kept him awake the previous night and whether the pain is constant. All patients with acute pain should be given an appointment on the day they call.

Staff meeting

In any discussion on communication, that between the dentist and staff must be considered a most important factor. Problems or difficulties encountered within the dental practice are usually found to have lack of communication as the root cause. Effective communication between the dentist and all staff is critical for the success of the practice and consequently for the positive motivation of its patients. For this reason, a meeting between the dentist and practice staff must be a regular feature. Such group communication is extremely time-efficient and productive. It helps to engender good team spirit and a sense of belonging to a group.

There are, however, a number of guidelines which should be followed to ensure that maximum benefit is derived from the staff meeting. These are:

- The meeting must be held regularly on a specific day and at a specific time. Most practices hold a meeting at least monthly but others feel it necessary to meet weekly or fortnightly. Whatever the frequency, a specific day and time must be decided upon which is most convenient for everyone.
- The meeting should not be held at a time outside normal working hours and certainly not at the end of a day. After a hard day's work, there is a tendency for both dentist and staff to want to get away as quickly as possible and a full discussion is therefore not always possible.
- When the timing of the meeting has been decided, the appropriate amount of time must be blocked off in all appointment books. Holding meetings during working hours will ensure maximum contribution from everyone.

- Every member of the practice should attend—dentists, hygienists, chairside and reception staff, and juniors.
- The practice manager or senior receptionist should act as secretary to organize the meeting and prepare an agenda.
- Every member of staff should be asked to put forward topics for discussion.
- The secretary must take brief minutes only of decisions taken at the meeting and these must then be followed up and progress reported at the next meeting. If this is not done, decisions tend to be forgotten and are therefore not acted upon.
- To achieve maximum benefit from the meeting, it is important to create an atmosphere which is informal and relaxed so that even the most junior members of staff feel they can put forward ideas and opinions constructively and in a friendly atmosphere.
- The subjects for discussion might include: ideas for practice improvement, identifying difficulties with fee collection, appointment scheduling, stock control and any problems which are impairing the efficiency of the practice. The emphasis must be on positive and constructive ideas.
- Discussion should be two-way. The meeting should not be used as a medium for the dentist to present a long list of complaints to the staff. The whole idea of a staff meeting is that everyone must feel part of the practice team and identify positively with it.

The meeting need not always be confined to discussion on administration. The need for staff education has been stressed previously and such meetings provide an ideal opportunity for this. To increase involvement even further, members of staff could be asked to prepare short papers or projects on a subject of dental interest.

3   Time management

Appointments

Correct appointment scheduling is the very basis of practice efficiency. A good appointment system will maximize productivity, minimize wastage of time, reduce tension and help the patient without causing the dentist to work inefficiently.

The appointment book

As the 'control centre' of the practice, this is the key to a smoothly running day, playing an important part in reducing practice pressures for dentist and staff and in this respect affecting their whole working existence. For these reasons, the design of the appointment book itself is most important. All dentists have individual preferences for the way in which their working day is organized and the design of the book must make allowance for this which permits the dentist to work in exactly the way he wishes.

Types of appointment book

Single column

The whole week is visible. This allows easy assessment of the workload for the week. Where there is more than one operator (whether a dentist and hygienist, or several dentists), a separate book is needed for each one. The main disadvantage of this type of book is that it takes up a great deal of working space when open on the reception desk. Where several books need to be used, an enormous area of desk top may be required if they are all left open. As most reception areas do not have this amount of space available, the books have to be closed and stored in pigeon-holes in front of the receptionist. This means the receptionist has constantly to take each book out and replace it when making appointments for the different operators.

Multiple column

Each day is ruled into two, three or four columns corresponding to the number of operators. It has the advantage that only one book needs to be kept open and thus the design is reasonably economical of space. Since books do not have to be taken out and replaced for appointments with different operators, pigeon-holes are not required. The disadvantage is that only two days are visible at a time and therefore the spread of the workload may not be as easy to assess.

Where space is very limited at the reception desk, the book can be placed on a single-tiered, long plinth, which should slope at an angle of approximately 45 degrees from the counter top to the working surface. This gives the correct angulation of the book for the receptionist to see and write on while leaving sufficient working space on the desk.

Time-management appointment system

This is suitable for a single or multiple operator. The current day only is displayed but the margins of subsequent days are also visible and show the appointment times for each day of the week. As appointments are made for subsequent days the times are crossed off—this shows at a glance what appointment days and times are available without turning pages for the week and gives a very clear indication of the workload for the operator. The design can be printed for single and multiple operators and its advantage is that only one book is required for up to four operators, with consequent saving of space.

Custom-made

Some companies customize appointment sheets to the dentist's own requirements. The dentist has first to decide on the starting and finishing times, time intervals and the number of columns per day, and the company prints the sheets and supplies a binder. They can be supplied dated or undated— the latter would be chosen by those dentists who prefer to date stamp the appointment sheets themselves (see page 32).

An alternative to having the sheets commercially printed is to print them on the practice computer, or to have them photocopied from a master copy designed by the dentist and drawn by a suitably artistic member of the staff. This is a very inexpensive method in that it reduces costs by eliminating printing but also allows for future changes in the appointment system. It is a relatively simple matter to amend or redraw the master copy and reduplicate.

Design of the appointment page

The ideal page should have:

- Short time intervals. Many books are divided into quarter-hour intervals and this limits the length of an appointment to multiples of 15 minutes only. Taken over a whole day this usually creates some loss of working time. This can be minimized by using 10-minute time intervals, which allows greater flexibility and more accurate and more efficient use of time.
- Space for the patient's name and the appointment time allotted.
- Adequate space for the type of treatment. This is essential for the information of both the dentist and the DA (see below).
- The lunch interval should be heavily blocked out so that no patients' names are written therein. It is most important that both the dentist and his staff have an adequate lunch break for rest and relaxation.
- A space for the 'buffer zone' (see below) and mid-morning and afternoon breaks if the practice requires these.

All these features can be most easily incorporated into a custom-printed appointment sheet.

Whichever design of appointment sheet is employed, all books should be loose-leaf, preferably in a ring-binder with as many rings as possible. This reduces sheet tear-out at the holes and makes the sheets much easier to turn over. Ideally pages should be taken out as they are used, so that only the current week is displayed when the book is opened. It eliminates the constant turning of pages when the appointments are being made. Used appointment sheets should be saved and stored as a record.

Making the appointment

Figure 3.1 shows the information which must be recorded for each patient.

Name, initials and sex

A full forename should be included if the patient's surname is a common one. This ensures that the correct card is taken out of the filing system. There can be nothing more frustrating than to have a patient in the dental chair ready for treatment and then to find that the record card is for the wrong patient. The consequent hiatus and waste of time while the correct card is found and brought into the treatment area causes tension for both the dentist and an already-tense and nervous patient.

Phone number

A daytime phone number should be obtained for all new patients so that they can be contacted if the appointment has to be changed or cancelled by the dentist. Even in the best organized office, sudden emergencies can occur (for example, the dentist may be taken ill). In such a case, failure to contact the patient and reschedule the appointment may well cause him considerable inconvenience and wastage of time and could even result in the patient leaving the practice.

Time

Time to be allotted for the appointment should be written in figures and the interval marked off with a definite line. The best indicator of appointment time is an arrow clearly defining the end of the appointment, since this is simple and accurate in apportioning the time. Indefinite demarcation or no demarcation at all usually results in the patient being given less appointment time than intended, due to other patients' names being entered into the space left in the book. Not only does this result in insufficient time being given to the patient first appointed, but it also places pressure on the dentist and his staff by overloading the treatment session.

Type of treatment

The type of treatment to be delivered at that appointment should be recorded. While this is obviously important for the dentist, it is also necessary for the DA so that she can pre-set and prepare instruments and materials and check that laboratory work has been returned.

Special information

Any special information about the patient should be indicated by marking the book with code letters against that patient's name:

H Patient scheduled to see the hygienist as well as the dentist. This ensures that both appointments are erased should the patient cancel. It also shows the dentist that he can see the patient for recall examination in the hygienist's room if this should be necessary.

NP New patient. The dentist would then know in advance that he must first talk to the patient in the consultation area.

AB Patient on antibiotic cover. This ensures that the dentist checks that the medication has been taken.

P Payment of fees overdue. If no fee has been paid at that visit, the dentist can discuss this with the patient before further treatment is given. Usually a personal word results in the overdue account being settled. Failing this, the dentist may want to give either very minimal treatment or in extreme cases no treatment at all.

E Emergency—patient in acute pain.

R Patient to be telephoned the day before the appointment with a reminder. This is particularly important if a long appointment has been allotted or if the patient has to take premedication or antibiotic cover. It is well worth the small amount of time and effort involved in making a phone call to prevent a possible broken appointment with consequent loss of time for the dentist or hygienist.

The buffer zone

Flexibility in the appointment book is essential for good timekeeping and a smoothly run day. It can only be achieved by the use of the *buffer zone*. This is a 30- or 40-minute space in the appointment book with a diagonal line drawn through it to indicate that no formal appointment must be scheduled in (see Figure 3.1). Depending on the wishes of the individual dentist and the patient flow through the practice, either a single buffer zone can be used or one placed in the morning and one in the afternoon.

Advantages

Late running

It absorbs late running and ensures that the morning and afternoon sessions are finished on time.

Emergencies

Emergencies can be appointed into the buffer zone and this allows the practice to offer the facility of treating patients in pain on the same day, without disrupting the appointed patients. It hardly needs to be emphasized that it is the dentist's moral duty to see patients in acute pain on the day in which they call the practice.

Ultra-short appointments

It can be used to make ultra-short appointments, for example removal of sutures, insertion of temporary dressings, and easing of restorations and dentures.

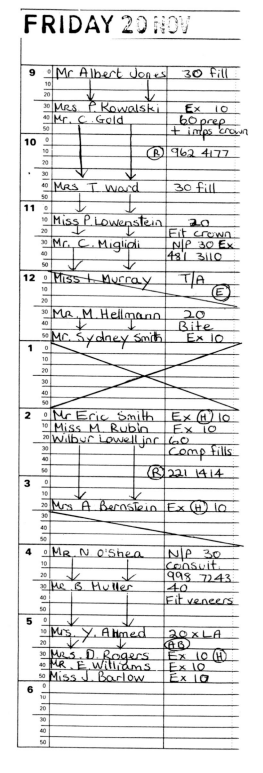

Full forename

Patient to be telephoned on previous day

New patient—contact telephone number

Emergency placed in buffer zone

Hygienist appointment with exam

Time clearly demarcated

Buffer zone

Type of treatment indicated

Antibiotic cover

Figure 3.1

Examples of correctly (this page) and incorrectly filled (opposite) appointment pages. A large stamp has been used to print each day and date. The code letters provide special information about individual patients (see page 31).

MON. 23rd OCT

No initial or forename	**9** 0	Mr Jones	30
	10	X X	
	20		
	30	Mr. M. Dyer	30 Fills
Time not blocked off	40		
	50		
	10 0	Miss G. Patel	
	10	Mrs. J. McLain	
	20		crown prep
	30		
	40		
	50	Miss D. Walkowski	
	11 0		Imps
	10		
	20		
	30	Larry W. Snyder	?
	40		
No telephone number for new patient	50	Miss I. Jackson	Ex N/P
	12 0	Mr. S. Grainger	Fill 30
	10		
	20		
	30	Miss M. Murphy	40
	40		
Treatment over-running into lunch hour	50		
	1 0		
	10		
	20		
	30		
	40		
	50		
	2 0	Miss S. Brown	Ex
	10		
	20	Mr. B. R. Grahame	Ex (H)
	30	Mr Kent	60
	40		Crown prep
	50		
	3 0		
	10	Mrs. P. Benson	Pain
	20		
	30	Mr R. Flanagan	Treat
Patient squeezed into existing appointment	40		
	50	Miss E. Brunner	Ex
	4 0	N. Jenkins	N/P
	10		
	20		
	30		
Time not clearly demarcated	40	Emilio Gavrotti	Fill 40
	50		
	5 0		
	10	Mr Hu Ying	Ex
	20	Mr Perry	Ex
Treatment not specified	30	Miss S. O'Neill	
	40		
	50	Fr S. Casey	Ex
	6 0		
	10		
	20		
	30		
	40		
	50		

Introductory appointments

New patients can be scheduled for a short introductory appointment if the dentist is fully booked a long way ahead. The opportunity to get the new patient into the practice at an early date will help to ensure that the patient remains with the practice. Even if little or no treatment is given at that appointment, a relationship is established between the dentist and the new patient on which future treatment can be built.

Telephone calls

All outgoing telephone calls from the dentist should be made during the time of the buffer zone. No incoming calls must be put through to the dentist while he is treating a patient and similarly the dentist must not make telephone calls at this time. To do so implies that he is not giving his full and undivided attention to the patient in the chair and is extremely poor for public relations.

All incoming calls for the dentist must be taken by the receptionist, and the caller's name, telephone number and the nature of the call recorded on a telephone message pad (see page 38). Assuming that the nature of the call is one which only the dentist himself can deal with, the caller should be informed that the dentist is with a patient and so unable to come to the telephone. The formula to use is: 'Mr X is with a patient at the moment. Please leave your number and he will call you back as soon as he is free.'

Relaxation

It is most important that the dentist and his staff have a 5- to 10-minute break in both the morning and the afternoon in which to relax. Dentistry is a very highly pressured profession and both the dentist and the patient suffer if such relaxation breaks are not taken.

The day sheet

A photocopy of the relevant appointment sheet for each day should be made. As an alternative to photocopying, some companies supply 'no carbon required' (NCR), or carbonless, appointment sheets which produce a duplicate for use as the day sheet. Whichever method is used, an *exact* copy of the day's appointment list must be produced, which is then posted in each treatment area and acts as the day sheet for each operator. This should be prepared during the early afternoon of the previous day to allow time for the DA to check that all laboratory work has been returned. This is the responsibility of each individual operator's DA. Should a piece of work not have been returned by the technician, he must be contacted immediately and the reason established. Should the technician then be unable to return the work in time for the appointment next day, the patient can be notified and given another appointment. There is nothing more calculated to produce annoyance, poor practice image, and indeed loss of a patient from the practice than for the patient to keep an appointment on the correct day and time only to find that the dentist cannot carry out the treatment because the technician has not completed the work.

It is also most important that the receptionist notifies those in the treatment area immediately of any changes in appointments so that the day sheet can be amended accordingly. A cancelled appointment may allow the dentist to do more work on the patient currently being treated, thus saving time for both. Conversely, if the receptionist schedules in an extra patient and forgets to inform staff in the treatment area, the dentist, working with the original day sheet, assumes that he has adequate time for the current patient and is subsequently placed under unnecessary pressure.

A further very important function of the day sheet is that, because it is an exact copy, the code letters entered into the appointment book are duplicated onto the day sheet, which thus gives the dentist an immediate note of any special patient information.

Common problems in appointment-making

Emergencies

Unless a Buffer Zone is used, these will interfere with appointment-scheduling.

Patients who are habitually late

One way of dealing with them is to make their appointment time in the book 10 minutes later than the time on their appointment card. This is not entirely without hazard because occasionally such a patient may turn up 'on time'.

Patients who fail appointments

There are several ways of minimizing failed appointments. The most effective is to remind the patient by telephone on the day prior to the appointment. This is particularly important for those patients with lengthy appointments and those scheduled for the hygienist, especially if this is coupled with a recall appointment for the dentist. It is well worth the time and trouble of making such a call if it ensures the attendance of a patient who may otherwise fail. It is also helpful to have a list of patients who live or work locally and who could come in at short notice.

Patients who do fail appointments must be telephoned as soon as the receptionist realises that the appointment is not being kept. This makes it immediately apparent to the patient that a dentist and a nurse are waiting for him and that their time has been wasted. A new appointment can then be made immediately. If there is a delay before telephoning the patient, the impact is lost and making a further appointment may be more difficult.

Many practices charge a fee for failure to attend but opinions differ on the effectiveness of this measure. Factors which have to be taken into account are that, to make it worthwhile, a patient would have to be charged an amount corresponding to the dentist's hourly work rate but the patient may consider such a fee exorbitant. In addition the patient may feel that on paying the fee he has absolved his guilt and may again fail appointments in the future. The financial advantage of charging must be balanced against the possibility of the patient feeling aggrieved and leaving the practice. Another factor which must be taken into account is the possible future treatment potential not only of that patient but also of the rest of his family. If a patient habitually fails appointments, there is a case for a face-to-face discussion with the

patient, who should be asked to decide whether he wishes to remain with the practice. Often in this way pressure can be brought on him to keep all future appointments.

In practical terms, the only solution for such patients is to make only single appointments of fairly short duration and to obtain a cash deposit on the first visit. This itself is often a factor in motivating future attendance.

Neither of these last two categories should be booked in at times which are popular with patients or at peak periods of the day.

No record in appointment book

The patient may arrive for an appointment which has been marked on the appointment card, although no record appears in the book. This can be avoided by making it an absolute rule that, when the appointment is made, the patient's name is written first in the book and then on the card. If the receptionist is under pressure, it is easy to make the error of writing the patient's appointment card, handing it to the patient and then forgetting to write the appointment in the book.

Mistaken attendance

If the patient arrives at the wrong time or on the wrong day, this can sometimes be the result of receptionist error but is usually because the patient has misread his appointment card or not read it at all. Needless to say these patients rarely have their appointment cards with them when they attend. Sometimes patients make mistakes because they have written the appointment in their own personal diary and the receptionist relies on this being correct and does not give them an appointment card. To preclude this possibility, *every* patient should be given an appointment card.

Appointment with wrong partner

In a group practice, the appointment may be written into the wrong book. Appointment books should be clearly colour coded and, in a large practice, even appointment book sheets may be different colours for each partner.

Patient swap

A patient may exchange his appointment with another member of his family, failing to realise that the treatment for both is totally different and has been allotted vastly different times. The solution is to inform the patient not only of the date and time of the next appointment but also of its duration. Where long appointments are involved, this should be written on the appointment card as well.

Single or multiple booking

Appointments for a prolonged course of treatment can be booked singly or as a series. Though the latter is usually more efficient in that treatment is completed over a shorter period of time, many patients tend to fail at least one of a series of appointments more readily than if they only had a single one booked. A balanced view must be taken of the points for and against each of the two methods and an individual judgment made, based on the dentist's assessment of the patient and his past record.

Methods of apportioning time

There are three types of appointment in terms of time requirement:

- Predictable—for example conservation, denture try-in, crown and bridge preparations and impressions, scaling.
- Unpredictable—for example oral surgery.
- Variable—the recall examination. The appointment time can be varied by either doing the examination only or, if work is necessary, beginning that work at the recall appointment should time allow. This is a good way of filling in space caused by cancellation or failed appointments.

Two methods commonly used to apportion time are estimation and application of a 'blueprint'.

Estimation

This is mostly employed for the predictable appointment. It uses the dentist's own experience to produce an accurate estimate of the time he would require for any given procedure, and takes into account the dentist's own assessment of the degree of difficulty of each individual case. It takes into consideration not only the clinical procedure but the temperament of individual patients.

Only the dentist himself should make the decision on the time to be allotted to the next appointment for any procedure. He must inform the DA of the time required and this instruction must be adhered to by the receptionist.

As this is only an estimate, it cannot always be totally accurate since unforeseen difficulties can occur from time to time. Over-running of appointments is therefore sometimes unavoidable, although, in general, most experienced dentists usually estimate with an amazingly high degree of accuracy.

However, there are dentists who prefer to eliminate the guesswork from appointment estimation and to establish accurate timings for every procedure. This should be done by arranging for a junior member of staff to be present in the treatment area for an entire week and, using a stopwatch, to time every type of procedure performed by the dentist. The times should all be noted down and an average can then be calculated. This may then be used by the dentist to make a more accurate assessment of the time he wishes to allow to procedures in the future. However, it must be emphasized that the other factors mentioned above must also be taken into account in individual cases.

The 'blueprint'

The 'blueprint' is the name given to an idea conceived by K Cooper of the UK. The practitioner draws up his own blueprint by grouping the different types of treatment into specific areas of the day. This blueprint is then identical for each day and every week. It gives a greater degree of organization of the week and of the appointment system, but is much more rigid. The advantage is that it allows the receptionist to tailor the day to the dentist's own personal wishes and preferred method of working. This presupposes that he has fixed ideas on the format of each day. For example, the dentist may prefer to do crown and bridge work in the first half of the morning, prosthetics at the end of the day and children in the early part of the day or after school hours. Many like to finish early on a specified day and prefer to see emergencies in the early morning or late afternoon. The dentist must discuss with the receptionist the type of day he sees as ideal and then implement this by formulating his own 'blueprint'.

Stages in 'blueprint' planning

- Every procedure must be timed accurately for one week.
- The receptionist checks through the previous 3 months' appointments to establish how many hours have been taken performing different general functions, for example conservation, *x* hours; prosthetics, *y* hours, etc.
- In conjunction with the dentist, the receptionist draws up a 'blueprint' of the ideal week, and all appointments must then only be scheduled at the times of day which are reserved for them.

The disadvantage of the 'blueprint' is that it is extremely rigid and does not take into account the difficulty some patients genuinely have in attending only at the specified part of the day allocated to that type of treatment.

Appointment planning

Even where a full blueprint is not rigidly applied, there should be a basic pattern in every appointment book. A great many dentists feel that they are earning their maximum potential when they are seeing the maximum number of patients. However, this is often counter-productive because a practitioner working under pressure and running late tends to do less actual work on each patient in order to relieve the pressure. In an ideal world, the most financially productive day would be produced by seeing one patient and working on that patient for the entire day. However this is rarely practical but it does mean that the pattern of appointment making must allow adequate spaces for long and

therefore more productive appointments. Short appointments such as recalls should not be spread throughout the entire day but grouped together into set periods to allow adequate facilities for long appointments to be made.

Communication between treatment area and reception

Although many practices are equipped with interroom telephone systems, it is important that these are not used to communicate to the receptionist details about the length and type of appointment for patients. Errors are frequently made when verbal communication is used and can only be eliminated by using written communication. One of the best ways to do this is by the use of a printed slip attached to each patient's record card. The following information is entered by the DA prior to the patient leaving the treatment area:

- Type of procedure to be undertaken at the future appointment(s).
- Length of time required for future appointment(s).
- If laboratory work is involved, the length of time to be allowed before the next appointment to ensure time for the work to be completed and returned.
- Any fee to be collected for the treatment given at this appointment.

The slip and record card are given to the patient who then presents it to the receptionist, so providing her with clear and accurate information with which to make the appointment. Only in this way will the correct length and type of appointment be made for the patient and errors eliminated. When the appointment has been made, the slip is removed from the card and disposed of.

The telephone and the receptionist

This is often the patient's first contact with the practice and telephone calls must be received in a courteous, friendly and helpful manner.

- The telephone must always be answered promptly in a pleasant voice, with the words: '...'s practice ... speaking. How may I help you?' It is said that if one smiles when answering the telephone it comes through into the voice.
- It should always be remembered that there is a live listener at the end of the telephone.
- Patients enjoy being recognized. For example 'Yes, Mr Jones. How may I help you?' gives the correct impression that he is an important patient of the practice.
- New patients should be asked for the name of the person recommending them.
- If the receptionist is busy attending to a patient when the telephone rings, she should announce the name of the practice and her own name, followed by: 'Please hold the line and I will attend to your call in a moment.' The patient on the other end of the telephone cannot see that the receptionist is busy so, if more than 15 seconds elapse, the receptionist must return to the caller to let him know that she is still busy with another patient. A caller must never be left holding a silent telephone as this can imply that the receptionist is ignoring him or has gone on holiday very suddenly! When the receptionist is free to deal with the caller, an apology should be given, for example 'I am sorry to have kept you waiting but now I am free. How may I help you?'
- The initial ire of an angry patient can often be mitigated by the receptionist giving him a little time to cool down. This is best effected by telling the patient that she will check his records and call him back. This provides a sufficient cooling off period. It also gives the receptionist a chance to look at the record to see what occurred on the last visit and discuss the matter with the dentist before getting back to the patient.
- All incoming calls to the dentist must be filtered off by the receptionist and details entered on a printed telephone message pad kept near the telephone as described on page 34. Details which must be recorded should include the date and time of the call, who the message is for, nature of the call (business or personal, urgent or non-urgent), the action required and, most importantly, the caller's name and telephone number. The person taking the call should initial the message.

- No fees, other than that for the initial consultation, should be quoted on the telephone. Any patient asking for a fee estimate must be told firmly that this will only be given after the dentist has seen him for a consultation and before any treatment is given.
- Patients must not be given too much leeway in making appointments; instead specific questions should be put to them, for example 'Do you prefer mornings or afternoons, early or late in the day?' Having established these basic facts, the receptionist can offer a precise day and time.
- The receptionist must always imply she is trying to help. Positive statements such as: 'We are giving you the first appointment we have' are preferable to negative ones such as: 'I am sorry, we are fully booked next week.'

The telephone questionnaire form

This is filled out whenever a new patient telephones the practice for the first time. The first contact from a new patient is nearly always via the telephone and such a form is an extremely useful aid to obtaining information from the patient and providing some preliminary background for the dentist (Figure 3.2). Apart from the name, address and both day and evening telephone numbers, the most important detail to elicit is whether the patient is attending for routine examination or because there is a specific problem. Where the patient is attending for treatment of acute pain, more specific questions should be included, to establish, for example, the duration, intensity and approximate location of the pain and whether any treatment has been sought elsewhere. The psychological effect for a new patient of discovering that the dentist knows about his personal dental problem is most impressive and makes the patient immediately feel that he is in a caring atmosphere.

At the end of the call, the patient should be informed that confirmation of the appointment will be sent through the post. This should be accompanied by a medical questionnaire and a copy of the practice brochure (see pages 13–14).

Appointment cards

These should reflect the practice image and as such can be very useful for public relations. They should

TELEPHONE QUESTIONNAIRE

1. NAME ....

2. DID ONE OF OUR PATIENTS RECOMMEND YOU? ....
3. TELEPHONE NUMBER DURING OFFICE HOURS
4. ARE YOU HAVING ANY DENTAL PAIN AT THE MOMENT? YES/NO.
5. IF SO, CAN I HAVE A FEW DETAILS SO THAT WE CAN ARRANGE A SUITABLE APPOINTMENT FOR YOU.

....

PAIN
6. IS THE PAIN CONTINUAL OR JUST OCCASIONAL?
7. DOES ANYTHING BRING THE PAIN ON: HOT OR COLD, EATING OR PRESSURE?
8. IS IT A FRONT OR BACK TOOTH?
9. DOES THE TOOTH APPEAR TO BE BADLY BROKEN DOWN AND IS THERE ANY SWELLING?

....

CROWN
10. IS IT BROKEN OR IN ONE PIECE?
11. IS IT FIXED ON A POST?

....

12. ANYTHING ELSE TO NOTE

....

WE CAN SEE YOU ON ....
IF I COULD HAVE YOUR ADDRESS, I WILL SEND YOU CONFIRMATION TOGETHER WITH SOME INFORMATION ABOUT THE PRACTICE AND A MEDICAL FORM THAT I WOULD LIKE YOU TO FILL OUT.

ADDRESS

APPOINTMENT AND MEDICAL FORM SENT [   ]

Figure 3.2

A telephone questionnaire form giving background information about a new patient.

therefore be distinctive and attractively designed, with a modern style of print face and wherever possible a practice logo. A light pastel-coloured background for the card is preferable. Brightly coloured eye-catching appointment cards have been shown to reduce the percentage of patients who forget to attend for appointments (Draycott, 1986). Use of a white card can be compensated for by attractive-coloured print. Many dentists now prefer the appointment card to be in the form of a small booklet which introduces the practice and the facilities offered to patients. This is fully described on pages 15–16.

Recall systems

In order to maintain an adequate patient flow throughout the year and ensure a sound patient basis for future years, a good recall system must be an integral part of every practice. This is important, however busy the dentist may be at a given moment (because this demand may not last indefinitely) and however motivated his patients are. The main methods of recall are by:

- Advance appointment
- Telephoned reminder
- Mailed reminder
- Mailed appointment

Advance appointment

This is made at the completion of a course of treatment. At the final visit, the patient is given a firm appointment for his recall examination before leaving the practice.

Advantages

- No cost involved.
- Minimal time spent by staff.
- Simple procedure.
- The appointment is written in the book so that, if the appointment is failed, the patient can be followed up.

Disadvantages

- Patients often cannot foresee future commitments (appointments are failed or cancelled).
- Dentists sometimes cannot foresee future commitments (appointments may have to be cancelled).
- Short recall appointments may be scattered throughout the book several months in advance and make it difficult to book long appointments.

Telephoned reminder

The patient's name and daytime telephone number are entered on a small index card and stored in a file divided into months. Every month the block of patients therein is telephoned and a specific recall appointment is made.

Alternatively, the monthly recall list can be incorporated in a computerized system or in a colour-coded filing system. Computerized recall is probably one of the most cost-effective methods (see pages 259–61). The colour-coded system is described more fully on page 44.

Advantages

- A more positive method.
- Immediate response more likely.
- Reduces likelihood of failed appointments.
- Cheaper—a phone call is much cheaper than the cost of printed stationery and postage.

Disadvantages

- Patients at work may be unable to come to the phone. The number may be busy or there may be no reply, necessitating more time spent in phoning again.
- Extremely time-consuming for the staff.
- Tendency for details of patients not contacted to get carried forward to the next month and to stack up.

Mailed reminder

The patient is sent a reminder requesting him to contact the office to arrange a recall examination.

Advantages

- Places responsibility on the patient.
- Patients always receive the card at their home even though they may not be contactable at work.

Disadvantages

- Patients ignore the request or overlook it and lose the card.
- Patients who do not respond are lost to the practice.
- Costly (postage plus printed card).
- Time-consuming for staff. However, this can be considerably reduced by patients addressing their recall envelopes at the end of each course of treatment.

Mailed appointment

The patient is sent a definite appointment time.

Advantages

- Good response.
- Patient's appointment is written in the book.
- If the patient does not keep the appointment, he will be registered as a failed appointment and can be followed up.

Disadvantages

- Extremely time-consuming for staff.
- Appointment book is heavily filled with recall appointments.
- Costly (postage, cost of printed card and staff time).

Recall time

There are three methods of allotting time for recall examinations. An appointment for the patient can be made:

- With the dentist only, for the recall examination.
- With the hygienist only.
- With both the dentist and the hygienist.

Recall examination appointment only

Advantage

Should the patient fail or cancel the appointment, only a small amount of time is wasted.

Disadvantage

The patient may travel a long distance for the appointment and may not appreciate having to re-attend for a second appointment to be treated by either the dentist or the hygienist.

Appointment with the hygienist only

In this case the recall examination is done by the dentist in the hygienist's room, once the appointment with the hygienist is complete.

Advantage

It ensures that, should the patient fail to attend, none of the dentist's time is wasted. His time is much more costly than that of the hygienist.

Disadvantages

The hygienist is under some pressure since she is prevented from seeing her next patient while the dentist occupies her room.

The dentist may have to leave his own patient during treatment when he moves into the hygienist's room to perform the examination. It may not always be convenient for the dentist to break off treatment and the patient he is treating may feel aggrieved that he is not being given the dentist's undivided attention.

Double appointment

In this alternative two appointments are made, one for the patient to see the hygienist followed by a short one for the dentist to perform the recall examination in his own treatment area.

Advantage

It is more convenient for the patient in that only one visit is required if no treatment is necessary.

Disadvantage

If the patient fails to attend or cancels the appointment, the time of both the dentist and the hygienist has been wasted.

Of these three alternatives, the one which is the most economical of the dentist's time is to make an appointment only with the hygienist and perform the examination in her room. However, the choice must be governed by individual patient's circumstances. For example a patient who travels a long distance *must* be given a double appointment, while one who has a history of persistently failing to attend should be given an examination appointment only.

Date stamps

Though rubber stamps of various types are used in the dental office, the simple date stamp can make the most valuable contribution to practice efficiency. The two major uses are on:

● The loose-leaf, undated appointment sheets (see Figure 3.1), for which a large date stamp should be used.
● Patient record cards, for which a small date stamp is necessary.

Date stamping appointment sheets

Advantages

● Saving of staff time.
● The appointment book can be rapidly stamped for several months ahead.

● Less likelihood of error than if written by hand.
● Public holidays and weekends need not be stamped, thus preventing the possibility of booking patients on these days, by mistake.

Date stamping patient record cards

Record cards should be taken from the file on the day before appointments, date stamped and placed in correct order in each treatment area together with the day sheet.

Advantages

● The DA's chairside time is saved because there is no need to write the date on every card.
● More accurate and prevents the possibility of the wrong date being written.
● Ensures that all treatment given at the appointment is written on the card. It is often possible to omit this vitally important step if chairside staff are under pressure or running behind schedule. Failure to record the treatment will be readily apparent to the reception staff because of the unfilled space against the date stamp and the card may then be returned for completion.
  Not only does omitting to write the treatment given contravene medical/legal guidelines but with no record of treatment no payment will ensue!
● If the patient fails to attend, it makes absolutely certain that this is recorded on the card, any omission again being noticed by the reception staff. This ensures that the patient's card is not refiled without the patient being contacted for a further appointment.

Filing systems

The heart of any professional office is its filing system. Efficiency rests on the ability to retrieve files easily and accurately, update them and return them quickly to the system without misfiling. Lost, misfiled or mislaid records can result in a good deal of stress for the dentist and considerably reduce practice efficiency. A filing system must be used which will eliminate this problem.

Methods of filing

Alphabetical

This is the conventional method and is open to a large number of errors. Cards take longer to file and retrieve than with the other methods and the possibility of misfiling is greatly increased, with consequent wastage of time.

Numerical

The index cards are numbered instead of being alphabetical. The record cards filed in each section are marked boldly in the top right-hand corner with the number of that section.

Colour coding

The best method of organizing a large filing system is by colour coding—the assignment of a colour to a number, letter or item to show meaning. People recognize colours and patterns of colour faster and at a greater distance than they do numbers or letters. By placing colours in position on a file folder, colour block patterns are formed. These blocks of colour speed searching time, save pre-sorting time and increase filing efficiency. Such a system reduces filing and retrieval time by up to 40 per cent.

Colour coding also makes misfiling impossible since mismatched colours readily show a file which has been misplaced.

There are two methods of assigning colour codes—alphabetical (alpha) and numerical. In both systems each file is assigned coloured labels which identify it as belong to a particular patient but which also code the file to make retrieval and refiling easier and more accurate.

Alpha filing

This is suitable for filing systems with up to 20 000 files. Two or three differently coloured alpha labels are applied to each patients' folder. The first label represents the first letter of the patient's last name. The second represents the second letter of his last name and third, optional, label represents the first letter of the patient's forename. Because each label is differently coloured, colour blocks form when the folder are filed alphabetically.

The labels can be arranged in two ways:

- Along the top of each folder if a vertical filing system is used.
- Along the edge of the file if an open-shelf (horizontal) filing system is used.

An additional label may be added to each file in either case indicating the year that the patient last attended for active treatment. These year labels can be used with both alpha and numerical systems and allow files of patients who have not attended for some years to be taken out of the file, thus providing extra space and preventing the filing system becoming clogged with inactive record cards.

The use of year labels also highlights patients who have missed their recall examinations and they can thus be followed up.

Numerical colour coding

Each folder is assigned a four- or five-digit number, the first number in the system being (0)0001. Such a system does require an alphabetical cross-reference file but is the simplest of all techniques to use and in fact the only practical one for offices with over 20 000 files.

Patients are allocated a specific number and the notes and record cards filed numerically. Members of one family may or may not be filed adjacently. A separate alphabetical index file or a simple computer database cross-links the patient to his code. A specific code number must then be used throughout the practice on letters, in the appointment book and on day lists. This assists the accurate and rapid retrieval of patients' records. If a patient rings to change an appointment for example, the receptionist can locate the record card within seconds.

Coloured tabs

Removable coloured metal tabs can be affixed to record cards when filed vertically, to denote the first letter of the patient's name, or to indicate the status of the patient in various categories. For example, colours can be chosen to indicate patients with a specific medical condition, patients in the middle of treatment but awaiting referral back from specialist treatment, patients owing money who have not been sent an account, patients who have been sent an account and patients who have failed appointments and require contacting. A small chart giving the key to the colour codes should be placed near the records.

A basic example is the use of the system in colour-coded recalls. A tab is placed in one of 12 positions along the top of the card to indicate the month in which the patient needs to be recalled. Each month all cards with a tab in that month's position are pulled and the patients recalled.

Card storage

There are two main methods of storing record cards: vertical and horizontal.

Vertical storage

A conventional floor-standing filing cabinet or a multi-tiered rotary file provides a means of vertical storage. Where space allows, the rotary file is preferable since it speeds up location and refiling. However, it requires a larger area than does the filing cabinet and is ideally more suitable for the large multi-operator office.

Horizontal storage

Either open-shelf wall-racks or a rotary file can be used, the former being much more economical of space. Open-shelf filing occupies only 25 per cent of the floor space required by filing cabinets and increases filing capacity by 300 per cent.

4   **Financial control**

The successful dental practice is the one that has tight control over its finances. There is absolutely no reason why such a practice should not be both ethical and commercially profitable. Unfortunately, a large number of dentists tend to undervalue their abilities, with the result that they do not charge fees which are consistent with their high level of skill and expertise. Their full earning potential is not realized. This obviously has a distinct effect on practice profits (or rather, lack of them).

Where fee levels are totally under the control of the dentist, he must first fix a realistic scale of fees for his services and then ensure that such fees are collected promptly.

Fee calculation

Dentists whose fees are paid either by the state (as under the National Health Service in the UK) or by private insurance schemes are paid a fixed fee per item, over which they have no direct control. However, dentists treating patients under private contract can set their fees at whatever level they wish and so must have a properly calculated scale of fees to apply.

Such a scale may be formulated on the basis of a fee per item of treatment, or an hourly rate may be applied.

Fee per item of treatment

Advantages

- It appears consistent to the patient.
- It is easy to calculate and apply.

Disadvantages

- For the patient: the fee might seem unacceptably high where several teeth are restored in one visit.

- For the dentist: this system fails to take into account the widely differing times required for the same procedure on different patients. For example, treatment of a large occlusal cavity in one patient may take three times as long as that of a minimal one in another, yet the fee is the same for both.

Hourly rate

This is calculated by directly relating the fee to the time spent on a procedure.

Advantages

- It is totally related to the degree of difficulty of the procedure.
- It is, therefore, fair to both the patient and the dentist.
- It encourages the dentist to spend whatever time is necessary to complete procedures to the highest possible standard. Time pressures are totally removed.
- Practice income is more predictable.

Table 4.1 Fee structure.

Fee per item
Examination
X-rays
Crowns, bridges, dentures
Endodontics
Hourly rate
Scaling and prophylaxis
Amalgam and composite fillings
Surgery
Paediatric dentistry

45

Table 4.2 Calculating hourly rates.

Gross receipts for previous year = G
Weeks worked per year = a
Actual chairside hours worked per week = b
Total chairside hours worked per year a × b = H

Hourly rate = $\dfrac{G}{H}$

Disadvantage

● It may be more difficult to calculate and apply.

The system used most widely in general practice is to combine a fee per item for predictable procedures (for example X-rays, crowns) with an hourly rate for non-predictable ones (for example fillings) (Table 4.1).

Method of calculating hourly rate

● Calculate the gross income received by each operator in that year (G).
● Calculate the number of chairside hours spent by each individual operator in the past year (H).
● Divide H into G and this will produce an hourly rate at which work was charged out for the past year.

Hourly rates must also be used in the calculation of fees for fixed items of treatment with related laboratory costs such as crowns, bridges and prostheses. The fee for such items would be based on the time involved (including both the preparation and fitting appointments) related to the hourly rate, plus laboratory and material costs. An additional percentage should then be added to allow for the higher skill factor involved in this type of procedure.

This rate must be examined and a decision made as to whether it is sufficient to produce the gross projected income necessary for the following year.

This must be related to the expected rate of inflation, estimated practice expenditure for the coming year, changed domestic circumstances (for example a new house, more children) and expected increase in practice costs and wages. Taking all these factors into account, it is possible to fix the desired hourly rate.

The next step is to draw up a table of the charge rates for fractions of an hour (see Table 4.3). Items having a fixed fee should be added to the list. Table 4.3 shows typical items for which rates should be calculated and listed. The table should be kept in the treatment area where it can be easily seen by

Table 4.3 Sample layout for fee scale.

Item	Fee	[Date]
Hourly rate items	*	
1 hour	*	
50 minutes	*	
45 minutes	*	
40 minutes	*	
30 minutes	*	
20 minutes	*	
10 minutes	*	
Fixed fee items	*	
Initial consultation (new patient)	*	
Recall examination	*	
X-rays—per film	*	
Scaling and prophylaxis (Hyg.)	*	
Crown	*	
Bonded	*	
Full gold	*	
Gold inlays	*	
One surface	*	
Two surface	*	
Three surface	*	
Porcelain jacket crown	*	
Porcelain post crown (1 cast post)	*	
Porcelain veneers	*	
Chrome partial denture	*	
Full dentures	*	
Rochette bridge	*	
Panorex	*	

both the dentist and the DA. It provides a form of ready reckoner and must be rigidly adhered to for every patient.

The table must be dated and the fee scale reviewed regularly. Ideally this should be done every 3 months, as this allows any rapid increases in inflation or practice expenses (in particular laboratory fees) to be compensated.

The use of a commercially produced ledger system allows practice profit to be monitored monthly and so allows fees to be adjusted more accurately. A small increase in fees every quarter is preferable to a large increase annually and may be more acceptable to patients.

Having such a written list of charges prevents the phenomenon, common in dentistry, known as 'mental–fiscal drag'. That is, in quoting a fee to a patient, the dentist has in mind the correct fee but in fact quotes a much smaller figure. It is said that this is often prompted by fear of rejection but there is also no doubt that dentists do not like to discuss money with patients. Reading a fee from a printed table helps to overcome this problem.

Application

The DA must note the time of the patient's entry and departure, and by reference to the fee chart can rapidly calculate the fee due for both hourly rate and fixed items, and enter it on the debit side of the treatment card and the operatory-to-reception slip. Alternatively the dentist himself can calculate and enter the fee. It is essential that this be entered on the card *before* the patient leaves the treatment area so that the information can be carried to the reception area for collection of the fee.

Fee collection

Perhaps the most vital component of the financially healthy practice is maintenance of good credit control—which, in effect, means the prompt collection of fees. However much work the dentist produces, it is of little account in the final analysis unless the fees for that work are paid to the dentist and paid promptly.

There seems to be no problem greater for dentists than that of collecting the fees due to them. There is an unfortunate tendency for dentists to apply the principle that patients should not be asked to pay anything until the complete course of treatment is finished. This can take a long time in complex cases and with a consequent effect on the cash flow of the practice.

Any treatment a dentist gives to a patient constitutes an article of value and, by not collecting the fee for that article, effectively the dentist is lending the patient the money equivalent to that fee.

It has to be pointed out that it is perfectly ethical to work on the simple basic principle that a patient should pay for treatment on the day that treatment is provided. This is unquestionably the best way of ensuring adequate cash flow as it eliminates slow payment or non-payment of fees.

Having stressed the need for applying a system whereby fees are collected at the end of every visit, it is essential that the reception staff apply this principle. One of the greatest problems to overcome is the diffidence which many staff (and most dentists) have of asking patients for money. There are a number of phrases which must *never* be used.

Forbidden phrases

- *You can pay next time*. This gives the patient a get-out that was not even asked for! Moreover, by the next visit, the patient will have forgotten

Table 4.4 Forbidden phrases.

You can pay next time.
We will bill you at the end.
I'm afraid it will cost . . .
Would you like to pay now?
I am sorry, there is . . . to pay.

how much care the dentist took, how much time he spent and how painless the procedure was. The old legal adage, 'Bill them while the tears of gratitude are in their eyes', is certainly one for the dentist to follow. It is quite likely that the patient would be perfectly willing to pay if only asked.

● *The secretary isn't here, why not leave your payment until next time.* This is simply another example of diffidence in asking for payment.

● *We will bill you at the end.* The patient's treatment may take several months to complete. If no fees are paid over this period, the dentist is earning nothing for that time. Moreover, should the patient leave the dentist before treatment has been completed, recovery of the fees accrued may be difficult, or even impossible. It only requires a few such patients to produce a marked effect on practice cash flow.

● *I'm afraid it will cost . . .* This implies the fee is very high for the service being rendered or equally may imply to the patient: *You may find this too expensive for your means.* Neither implication is acceptable.

● *There is . . . to pay—would you like to pay now?* Few people like to pay money at any time and a dental patient is no exception. This phrase implies to patients that they have a choice—and they usually take the choice to pay later.

● *I am sorry, there is . . . to pay.* There is no reason why either the dentist or his staff should be sorry to charge a patient for a service rendered with skill and care. The patient has been given a benefit and should expect to pay for it in precisely the same way as he would if he bought an article in a store.

The correct expression is: *There is . . . to pay today.* This makes a clear and unequivocal statement of fact and leaves the patient under no illusion of the amount of the fee and that it is payable immediately.

It is helpful to print the phrase in large letters on a card pinned behind the reception desk in direct view of the receptionist, though not of the patient. Visual stimulation is often conducive to verbal communication and the correct phrase is more likely to be used if the speaker is able to read it.

Reinforcement can be given by placing a suitable notice in the waiting room to the effect that fees are payable on each appointment unless prior financial arrangements have been made, for example:

'In order to keep practice expenses and therefore fee increases to a minimum, accounts will henceforth be rendered at each visit and your cooperation in settling these at the end of each appointment (in the absence of prior financial arrangements) will be much appreciated.'

A number of such notices are obtainable from dental office suppliers. If preferred, the dentist can have a notice designed with his own choice of wording. However, it must be properly printed and attractively framed.

Methods of payment

There are a number of different methods of payment:

● Conventional
● Cash discount
● Extended payment
● Credit card
● Banker's order

Whichever method is chosen, a clear decision must be taken at the initial consultation visit and an appropriate written agreement signed by both parties.

Conventional

Payment is made at each appointment for the full amount due for the treatment given on that day.

Discount

Where the patient is to have an extended course of treatment and has accepted the treatment plan, a 'courtesy' or 'early payment' discount may be offered for payment of the *total* estimated amount for the course of treatment *before* treatment actually begins, or at the first appointment where treatment is given. This has a dual advantage. The patient appreciates the reduction in total fee while the dentist receives a substantial fee before complete treatment is given and before laboratory fees are invoiced.

Extended payment

A deposit of at least one-third of the total fee is paid at the first visit, the balance being paid over a specified number of visits, depending on the length of the course of treatment. Should the complete treatment take only two visits, then a deposit of at least 50 per cent of the total fee must be paid at the first visit and the balance paid at the second one.

Where an extended payment arrangement has been made and payments are not paid promptly, a finance charge should be added, but the patient must be clearly informed that this charge is being levied. Usually, however, no finance charge is imposed on amounts paid in full within 21 days of receipt of the account for the instalment due.

Credit card

This is an ideal method of payment for large sums and may induce the patient to pay the full fee in advance. The advantage is that the credit-card counterfoil is a cheque which can be banked immediately and payment is guaranteed by the credit company.

Banker's order

This is a useful and acceptable method of payment for costly treatment. An initial deposit of at least one-third of the total fee is paid at the first visit, and a standing order arranged by the patient for monthly payments to be paid direct from his own bank account into that of the practice.

Patients may sometimes reject a costly treatment plan purely on financial grounds because they would find it difficult to raise immediate finance for the treatment. The extended payment, credit card and banker's order methods all allow patients to spread the cost over a period of time and for this reason they may well accept a treatment plan which they would otherwise have rejected.

The role of staff

It is the responsibility of reception office staff to collect all fees promptly at each visit but, if they are to do this, they must be given a clear indication from the treatment area of the amount payable for that particular visit. This information may be transmitted using one of the following:

● Patient record card
● Pegboard transaction slip
● 'Operator-to-reception' slip

Record card

The amount should be entered into the debit column of the record card. There are many record cards available which have columns for treatment delivered, charges and payments made. The DA should complete the record card in the treatment area, entering the treatment delivered and the fee to be debited for that visit. The patient then takes it directly to the receptionist. This has the advantage not only of clearly indicating the amount to be paid but also of allowing the receptionist to complete the card by entering the payment into the credit column. This saves having to complete the card at a later stage in the day—a task she may well forget. There is nothing more embarrassing and harmful to a practice image than to bill patients for amounts already paid, because of failure to maintain up-to-date records.

Pegboard transaction slip

The pegboard transaction slip (see later in this chapter) is extremely rapid to complete in the treatment area and a considerable time-saver for a busy chairside DA. As all transactions are subsequently recorded onto a ledger card by the receptionist, there is no possibility that the problem of omission described above will occur.

'Operator-to-reception' slip

The 'operator-to-reception' slip (see page 37) is completed with the amount payable for the treatment just rendered. The disadvantages of this method are that the DA has to write the amount twice—on the record card and on the slip—and it does not give the opportunity for the receptionist to enter payments made onto the card. It should therefore only be used if pegboard accounting is not employed and where the record card needs to be retained in the treatment area for some particular reason.

Treatment summary

Where a written treatment plan with an estimate of cost is not involved (see pages 23–4), and where treatment, though routine, is prolonged and involves a large number of visits, patients tend to forget the number of visits they have made and the actual amount of treatment they have received. A simple treatment summary is often helpful to act as a reminder and is an aid to good public relations. It gives treatment dates, an analysis of all the treatment delivered, and the fee chargeable to each. The summary may be given to the patient on completion of the course of treatment.

Summary forms can be obtained commercially or the dentist can have his own designed and printed to suit the individual type of practice.

Billing and collecting fees

Keeping records of transactions is a tedious and time-consuming process. Separate entries must be made on record cards and in the ledger, invoices written, day sheets entered and envelopes addressed. This repetition can be eliminated by the use of a 'one-write' (pegboard) system.

The one-write system

Advantages

- Eliminates repetition, thereby increasing efficiency

- Always accurate and up to date
- Provides a breakdown of treatment given
- Provides information for insurance claims
- Reduces the amount of cash owing by patients
- Improves cash flow
- Reduces costs

Components

- Accounting board
- Day-sheet record of charges and money received
- Transaction slips
- Patient's statement card

The day sheet and transaction slip are mounted on the accounting board and the statement card for the patient is inserted underneath.

Transaction slip

The transaction slip can be printed with the dentist's own name, address and logo and a list of the codes of the treatment which are provided. It is perforated into two sections: receipt/statement and stub. Arranged over a carbon strip are sections for date, description of the procedure completed at the appointment, the fee due, payments made and the balance due which make up the receipt/statement section of the slip. There is also space for the patient's next appointment. The transaction slip can be modified to contain additional information needed for insurance companies. When the slip is placed over the patient's statement card, details of any transactions are automatically transferred to that card.

The stub section serves as a communicating form between the dentist and the receptionist. It lists the patient's name, any previous balance outstanding, treatment codes and there is space in which the dentist can indicate the treatment given and timing and duration of the patient's next appointment. This stub section is attached to the patient's record card while the receipt/statement section is retained by the receptionist.

Using the system

Before treatment:

- The receptionist writes the patient's name and any balance of fee on the stub section.

- The stub is separated and attached to the record card, both of which are transmitted to the dentist. The receipt/statement section remains on the board.

After treatment:

- The dentist fills in the stub section indicating treatment given, fee due for this appointment and the timing and duration of the next appointment.
- The dentist gives the stub to the patient with instructions to present it to the receptionist.
- The receptionist places the patient's statement card under the receipt/statement section and transfers the information from the stub onto this portion of the slip.
- The receptionist informs the patient of the total fee due (including any outstanding balances). This usually prompts the patient to pay all or part of the fee at this time.
- The receptionist records the payment made by the patient. She then enters the next appointment and gives the receipt/statement section to the patient. This therefore acts as both a receipt and an appointment card and so saves expenditure on printing of both of these items.

In this way, the statement card is continually being updated and can be photocopied and sent off to the patient as a monthly statement of account if necessary. It has the advantages of showing the precise state of the patient's account to both the dentist and the patient. When completed, the statement cards are filed in a separate file.

Payment of practice accounts

The use of a one-write (pegboard) system for the payment of practice accounts has the advantages of:

- Ease of operation.
- Reducing clerical time.
- Increasing the accuracy of recording transactions.
- Reducing audit time by the accountants since one writing of a cheque produces duplicate details in the ledger for analysis. There is therefore no need to keep separate ledgers.

- The facility to prove accounts daily, weekly or monthly. The financial state of the practice is thereby kept completely under control at all times.

The system comprises printed cheques which carry the name, address and logo of the practice and which make carbonless duplicates. The accounting board is first loaded with a journal analysis sheet over which the blocks of cheques are clipped. The sheet has spaces for transaction details and 15 columns for analysis with an extra 9 optional columns if required on the other side of the sheet. There is also a section to record bankings made. All cheques have a remittance advice section which can be sent with the cheque and shows details of discount and of the number and amount of the invoices included in that statement. When the cheque is written, it copies directly through onto the journal sheet and it takes seconds to analyze the transaction after the cheque has been written.

The journal sheet can be checked either daily or weekly and it is possible to see at a glance the current balance by deducting payments made from deposits.

If necessary, the system can also be used for payment of wages by using specially designed journal sheets.

Stock control

Careful control of stock of consumable materials held is an essential part of good financial control. Over-stocking represents unnecessary expenditure and results in the tying up of working capital. The level of stock held must be no more than the minimum required to ensure that the practice will function efficiently at all times. A good stock-control system is one using T-cards—so called because of their shape.

Stock of all consumable materials should be placed, preferably in alphabetical order, on open shelves, labelled with the name of each item and the minimum amount of material which has to be maintained in stock. This provides a readily-assessed indication of stock levels. Every item should be given a T-card bearing its name. Cards can be colour-coded to group together types of consumable items such as impression materials, burs, linings and endodontic instruments. The cards can be filed in a special wall-rack.

When an item is ordered, the quantity and date of ordering are entered on the appropriate T-card, which is then filed in the extreme right-hand column of the rack. When the stock item is supplied, the date is entered on the card, which is then replaced into its original position.

All stock ordering and control should be placed in the hands of one specifically delegated member of the dental staff. To ensure that the exact item of stock ordered is supplied by the dealer, she must always ensure that the stock order form contains the full name of the item, size, manufacturer's name and correct unit of supply. For example, when burs are ordered, it must be clearly indicated whether they are to be high or low speed, diamond or tungsten carbide, right angle or straight, and their size and shape must be specified.

5 Computers in dental practice

Anthony S Kravitz BDS

In private practice, Manchester.

Until just a few years ago, the use of a computer was felt to be somewhat of a luxury and too complex for most small businesses. But, in the coming years, it is likely that computers will be as indispensable to general dental practitioners as the high-speed drill. This chapter is intended to aid practitioners in deciding about those parts of their businesses for which computers are required and what type of computer to obtain. Basically, when planning a purchase, one should always keep in mind the difference between features and benefits—money should not be spent on a feature highlighted by a salesman, which may derive no benefit to the practitioner.

This chapter is written to assist a wide readership—both those who know little about computers and those who are already computer-literate. Thus, the introduction explains the basics of computer hardware and later sections discuss 'software' and 'applications'. A glossary is given at the end of the chapter.

Introduction

A computer is a combination of a storage system and a calculator. The storage is a form of electronic record keeping, with information stored for use in a number of ways. Electrical charges operate on silicon chips, so that positive or negative charges turn microswitches 'on' or 'off' in an infinite array of combinations.

The computer consists of 'hardware', which is what one can see and touch (the machinery and wiring) and 'software', the part which makes the hardware work.

Hardware includes:

- central processing unit (CPU)
- input unit, such as a keyboard, mouse, light pen or scanner
- diskdrive(s)
- monitor, also known as a VDU (UK) or VDT (USA)
- printer
- modem
- wiring and cables to link the parts

Just as a car requires two essential components to make it work—a set of controls for the engine and the intelligence of a driver to use these controls in a meaningful manner—the **software** which makes a computer work comprises two components. There is an 'operating system' which controls the computer and 'applications software' which combines the operating instructions to produce a specific result.

Hardware

The hardware discussed here relates to personal computers (PCs or microcomputers). It is unlikely that many dentists would wish to install larger systems as a first-time purchase, in view of the small difference in power or facilities, although there is a large difference in cost between PCs and larger systems (minicomputers). As most dentists are likely to use the IBM-PC, or its compatible models, discussion is restricted to those systems.

Hardware comprises several components and dentists can mix and match these to suit their

53

requirements, provided always that they are compatible.

Central processing unit

At the heart of the machine is the central processing unit (CPU), also known as the microprocessor, which controls everything. The speed at which the CPU runs is very important, as a practitioner may want to process records for thousands of patients. The faster the speed of the CPU, the quicker the information will be processed.

The original IBM-PC CPU ran at 4.77 MHz. Faster speeds are now more usual and many machines are available with CPUs of 16–33 MHz (approximately ten times the original IBM speed), with little increase in cost. CPUs with even faster speeds are available, based on 386 and 486 'chips'. It must be appreciated that the jump from the simpler to the more complex microprocessors increases the cost of the hardware quite considerably. Individual advice should be taken on whether this extra cost is justified, following evaluation prior to purchase of hardware and software for the practice. Put simply, the larger the practice or more complex the software being operated in the system, the faster should be the CPU. For example, for a system utilizing word processing and desktop publishing (DTP) only (see page 58), a fast CPU would be unnecessary as the processing task involved is relatively simple.

Input units

As with all hardware, there are various complexities of **keyboard** available. The simplest comprise a typewriter-style keyboard with one or two additional keys to operate programs, such as 'control' or 'alt' keys. Typically they also have keys to operate the 'cursor' (pointer) on the screen and will usually have up to twelve function keys. These keys perform certain prescribed functions, which would normally otherwise take several key strokes. There may also be other keys, such as a separate numeric key pad (similar to a calculator keyboard) and other specialized functions keys.

Different types of input devices have been developed, such as the 'mouse', scanner and light pen. Usually these are in addition to the keyboard.

A **mouse** is a roller or optical device which moves the cursor around the screen and then performs individual functions when pressed onto a flat surface. Most programs available do not require the use of a mouse, as a keyboard is sufficient, but certainly for some specialized uses, such as desktop publishing, a mouse is a very valuable extra tool.

A **scanner** is a hand-held device which can be passed over text or photographs and which converts the shades of colour into dots of various intensity to be displayed on the monitor (see below). Subsequently, the information can be stored by the computer as part of data storage. This system is very useful for integration with DTP systems so that, for example, photographs or original articles can be read into a computer for later use or editing in a newly written article.

Light pens are simply that—they are similar to scanners but are usually used to read data from bar codes. They may be used in some applications to replace multiple keystrokes, much like a mouse.

Monitors

In Europe, monitors are also known as visual display units (VDUs) and, in the United States, as video display terminals (VDTs). Originally, monitors were only available with a very fuzzy black and white, white and black, green and black or amber and black picture (all known as monochrome or 'mono'). For most business uses, any of these types of monitor may be satisfactory if text only is going to be processed and if the operator is going to sit in front of the screen for not more than a couple of hours at a time. Colour monitors have been developed, available at increased cost, which may be visually more effective and relaxing for the eyes.

Graphics cards

Some programs require the use of graphics and, for this reason, a 'card' to run the graphics programs has to be installed into the computer. Typical graphics cards give an enhanced screen display by means of an increase in the number of dots (pixels) which make up the picture. This gives a sharper image, which is necessary for graphics programs. A dentist who is considering the use of dental charting on his computer would normally need to have installed such an 'enhanced graphics adapter', and a better quality monitor for the display of characters.

For just a small additional cost, monitors based on a video graphics array (VGA) card system are available. The picture quality produced by these systems can be compared to the quality of a colour transparency. Again, their use is particularly sensible for DTP packages.

Memory and data storage

All the above merely describes the hardware to work the computer. However, without 'memory', everything would be lost as soon as the machine was switched off. Thus, all machines need 'memory' or storage of information. The memory has two components. Firstly, the 'read only memory' (ROM), which comprises that part of the system which serves as a control for the computer. This cannot be altered normally by the user. Secondly, there is also the 'random access memory' (RAM). The RAM is the part of the system which holds all the 'applications' programs and data at any one time and the larger this memory, the quicker the machine will operate, whatever the CPU speed. A correct decision about the size of the RAM is relatively important, prior to purchase of the machine. However, if a RAM is purchased that is too small, it is possible with most machines to increase the size subsequently.

The usual operating system for PCs is MS-DOS (see page 57), or its derivatives. These systems are normally incapable of using more than 640K (approximately 640,000 characters of information – letters or numbers) in the memory at one time, thus most cheaper PCs are supplied with only this amount of RAM. For 'memory-hungry' programs such as spreadsheets, there are ways around this limit. Specialized memory cards are available which

redefine the way the operating system works. The more powerful 386 and 486-based machines use procedures to break through this barrier. Operating systems run by these CPUs therefore are not limited by this barrier.

RAM is transient and works only when the machine is switched on. Thus computers need some method of permanent storage of information—a 'filing cabinet' to store records. This is normally provided by disks in disk drives.

Disk drives

There are several different ways in which computers can store information permanently but, for the moment, PCs have only two practical ones—'hard' or 'floppy' disks (floppy disks are in fact small hard disks). These disks slot into 'drives'. All PCs have at least one floppy disk drive. Older technology machines, such as the original IBM-PCs, have 5.25 inch disks, which are 360K (approximately 360,000 characters of information). This is sufficient for the dental practice where wordprocessing only is being used. Modern machines have 3.5 inch disks with the data more closely packed, therefore holding anything up to 1.4 megabytes (1.4 MB) of information (1MB is 1,000,000 characters). Business-purpose computers would also have a second drive, either another similar floppy disk drive, or more usually a hard disk. The storage capacity of the latter could be anything from 20MB to 140MB. It is also possible to buy machines with two floppy disk drives, then add the hard disk later, either internally, in place of one of the floppies (where it will not be seen), or externally.

There are two fundamental considerations in the choice of disk. Firstly, for operating a business, a hard disk is always recommended. Floppy disks hold only limited amounts of data and therefore increased storage capacity as the business grows larger may be inhibited by the need to change floppies frequently. Hard disks also tend to be much faster in retrieving data from storage.

Secondly the largest size of hard disk that one can afford is also recommended. Certainly, most dentists with average-sized practices should have 40 MB or more. Information is stored as 'records' in files, and the files are spread randomly, in clusters, over the surface of the disk. Part of the disk is reserved by the computer for an index, the file allocation table (FAT), which tells the computer where to look for the files. Just as it is easier to file and retrieve record cards in a filing cabinet that is not too full, so the computer will work more efficiently with a larger disk.

Computers tend to be very reliable (see pages 63–4) but, for a number of reasons, it is possible to lose all the stored information. Hard disks do fail sometimes (known as 'disk crash'). They are not usually repaired on site but are replaced by the service engineer and repaired at a later date. This may mean that all the data stored on the disk is lost.

Back-up devices

Because of the possible failure of a hard disk, it is essential to have some kind of 'back-up' system, where a copy of the data can be made and kept separately. The data may then be taken from the premises for added security against fire or theft. Many businesses back-up their data to floppy disks, which is inexpensive as it only involves the purchase of two sets of disks. A foolproof arrangement for data security should always be made.

Unfortunately, while being inexpensive, backing up large amounts of data to floppy disks can be time consuming. It may take half an hour to back-up an average-sized hard disk and may require someone to supervise the process throughout. Other back-up systems are becoming much more widespread, as costs are reduced. Internal or external tape streamers can be installed which, with the correct software, can carry out the task in minutes. The small tape can then be slipped into the pocket, which is far more convenient than carrying a box of disks. These machines can be obtained at relatively low cost, but the special tapes needed can be costly.

Printers

The information displayed on a monitor is transient, as it is visible only when the computer is switched on. There is a practical need to have a printer in order to make 'hard copy' of the data, for example, to communicate with patients. Currently, there are three types of printers available:

- laser
- daisywheel
- dot matrix

Laser printers produce very high quality print, similar to that found in typeset publications. They may be used also as photocopiers. Their prime use is in desktop publishing (see page 58). However, they have a number of disadvantages, including their inability to produce output on continuous paper (for example, to print long lists) or on raised stationery, such as mailing labels. Their price is relatively high, and their speed low. Laser printers may therefore be inappropriate for the first-time user of computers.

To obtain a very high quality printing, it was formerly necessary to install a **daisywheel** printer. This can be described as similar to a typewriter plugged into the computer. Indeed, many of the currently available electric typewriters also have computer interfaces allowing them to reproduce computer output. The main disadvantages of daisywheel printers are their speed—they can be very slow—and their expense. Also, they too are not suitable for list printing on continuous roll stationery.

In dental practice, the most suitable choice is the **dot matrix** printer. Characters are made of little dots of ink impressed on the paper by rows of pins. The better quality printer gives dots closer together and thereby improved printing quality. In fact, many versions now have 24 pins, instead of the old 9-pin style, and printer controls enable them to produce 'letter quality' printing with little reduction in speed. The current generation of 24-pin printers may produce output in different styles (fonts) almost as good as laser print.

Other advantages of dot matrix printers include the possibility of sheet feeding or sprocket feeding. With sprocket feeding, the sheets are fed through the printer in one continuous roll which is not easily displaced as it is fed through on fixed sprockets (rather like film through a camera). Certainly for lists, this type of sheet feeding is more practical. Paper is available with perforated sprocket holes that can be torn away neatly.

The advantages of using a computer to communicate with patients make it essential for dentists to buy a good quality dot matrix printer. It would be wise, also, to have a less costly standby machine for use if, or when, the main printer breaks down.

Modems

Apart from printing, it is also possible to communicate using the computer by means of telephone lines. The main method of communication in which many dentists are now becoming interested is computer to computer.

In order to be able to send data from a PC, a modem is necessary. This converts the output of the computer into a meaningful code which is transmitted down a telephone line. External modems are available in the form of a small box, about the size of a telephone answering machine. Internal modems are available in card form. The speed of transmission both to and from the other machine will depend on the speed of the modem. Faster modems tend to be more expensive. Certainly for use in dental practice, a modem with a slow transmission rate is not recommended. A modem with a minimum 'protocol' of V22 (a speed of 1200/1200 Baud) is recommended.

Telephone lines are often of poor quality and degradation of the transmission can occur, so that the information received at the other end is not accurate. With modems for use other than access to public information systems, the extra cost of 'error correcting' machines should be considered as worthwhile.

Software

Introduction

It is the choice of software, or rather what the practitioner expects the computer to do for his practice, which is the most important initial decision in the purchase of a computer. Practitioners who are contemplating the benefits of computer installation should sit down and think through a careful evaluation of the planned uses. If an area of practice administration is not problematical, the use of a computer to run it may not be of any advantage.

Specialist programs should be suited to their purpose. For example, if one had decided to set up a specialist orthodontic practice then the latest gadgets which are available for endodontic therapy would be an unlikely purchase, even though they might be first-class for their purpose.

There can be little doubt, however, that most practitioners would benefit from the aid of a wordprocessor, as most dentists have to write letters frequently, many of which include similar or common phrases. The wordprocessor can help with this repetitive letter writing. At this point, it would be useful to give a brief description of the elements that comprise software and how software can be used.

Operating systems

There are several operating systems available for PCs, but it is reasonable to claim that MS-DOS (MicroSoft Disk Operating System) has become the world standard. This system has been regularly updated since it was first released in the early 1980s (see page 62). IBM PC-DOS is a compatible derivative of MS-DOS. Both are normally referred to just as 'DOS'. It is widely believed that approximately 90 per cent of all **applications** software currently available has been written to work using DOS **operating** software. Any would-be purchaser should hesitate to buy a computer which operates from a non-standard system, as this may limit the choice of available software. It is important for the hardware to be marked 'IBM-' or 'MS-DOS-compatible' as this indicates that it will almost certainly operate most software. Some 'clones' (machines that are cheap copies of IBM-compatibles) may not run all MS-DOS software. Similarly, before purchase of software, it is important to establish that it will run on the hardware in use.

However, MS-DOS does have limitations, and another operating system, OS/2, is now available, which operates differently. For example, it will allow the CPU to carry out 'multi-tasking' (performing different operations simultaneously). An OS/2-based machine will also operate DOS. Another increasingly popular operating system is Unix, which is suitable for networked applications (see page 59).

However, the volume of DOS software which is now available is so great that it is almost certain that any dentist who buys a computer operating from DOS will have machinery that is unlikely to go out of date for several years. Many suppliers, furthermore, have produced program enhancers to overcome the performance limitations of DOS. These include graphics programs which are pictorial menus and which use simulations and icons to facilitate program choice.

Applications software

There are now several different types of applications software available, including:

- wordprocessing
- spreadsheets
- communications
- graphics
- databases

Wordprocessing

Wordprocessing (WP) may be described as a method of manipulation of text. It is the one area of computerization from which every dentist, in general or other practice, would derive major benefits. A wordprocessor assists in more than just letter writing. It can be used for many purposes, including:

- clinical reports
- patient information leaflets
- 'in-house' typesetting for letter headings account forms, appointment sheets, etc
- customized appointment book sheets
- committee meeting minutes
- magazine and journal articles

Most WP packages include an automatic spelling checker and thesaurus.

There is an enormous range of WP programs available, at costs that vary depending upon the level of sophistication. One should choose a computer which will perform whatever other prime functions are needed in the practice and then purchase the word processor programs as an 'extra'. There is no need to spend vast sums of money to obtain WP software, as many of the less costly programs will do enough for most GPs. It would be foolish to obtain what is known as a 'dedicated' wordprocessor, which allows very limited database (see page 59) or spreadsheet (see below) functions. A dedicated program is one that performs the functions of that particular type of software only, perhaps to a higher functional ability than many users require.

Recent developments allied to WP have included the introduction of 'desktop publishing' (DTP). DTP is an exciting extension of WP. These programs allow the integration of text and graphics into one program, for the production of output such as newsletters, for example, in columnar form, as found in newspapers. The manipulation of printer letter styles is built into the program instructions to a greater extent than normal WP packages. In dentistry, these programs permit the production of very high quality practice leaflets/newsletters using modestly priced software packages.

The combination of WP and DTP, together with a reasonably priced printer and a photocopier opens up the possibility of a vast marketing strategy, relatively cheaply.

Spreadsheets

A spreadsheet is a program for the storing and manipulation of tables of information, usually numbers. Calculations can be performed automatically on the information, carried in specific sections of the tables, using pre-defined formulae. Good spreadsheets include simple graphing capabilities, which immediately enable the visually effective presentation of figures.

The use of spreadsheets is primarily in financial planning and historical analysis, which can assist in cash flow forecasts. Regular reports on profitability may be derived from information regarding income and expenditure. Many dentists like to carry out a monthly survey of their profit situation and a spreadsheet is almost certainly the quickest way to do this. A common problem with practice finance is that many dentists cannot afford to use accountants for financial planning. The dentist may complete the financial year and only later discuss the accounts in depth with the accountant, often after a few months. It may then be too late to undertake any reparative action recommended by the accountant.

However, the real advantage of a spreadsheet is the 'what if . . . . ?' ability of the program. Having identified an area of potential benefit or difficulty, one can instruct the computer to calculate the result of a change of circumstances in that area. For example, it is possible to analyse the final effects of the introduction of a new associate to the practice, or the profit forecast from the effects of inflation at various percentages on different parts of income and expenditure.

Communications

Until recently, communications software was probably not of great relevance for dental practitioners, as few dentists had the hardware capable of communication via the computer. Furthermore, public 'databases' which could be accessed by computer did not carry a great deal of interesting or useful information for running a small business. Recently, things have changed markedly and, in many countries, networks linking various aspects of health work are being developed.

However, standard specifications have had to be produced so that different computers can understand one another. The communications software has to be able to translate the output from the transmitting computer into a meaningful form to be sent down telephone lines to the receiving computer. Fortunately, most communications software available is relatively inexpensive and may be included in the price of a modem.

Communications is becoming a more integral part of dental business, in ways other than dentist to dentist. For example, most banks are now offering modem links to customers' accounts and it is possible to carry out advanced financial transactions using PIN numbers and PCs. Furthermore, where a substantial income is to be claimed by

dentists from third parties, such as insurance companies or government agencies, there is a large increase in the use of modem links for payment claim, as the process is greatly accelerated.

Finally, it is important to mention **networking**, that is, when two or more computers are linked to operate together (rather than just for the transfer of data). Special communications software is needed for the more sophisticated functions required (for example, file locking—the prevention of two users trying to access and edit the same data concurrently). Networking may involve more expensive applications software also, and a first-time user would be wise to consider very carefully before starting with a networked system, unless professional advice and experience are freely available.

Graphics

Graphics software permit graphs, bar and pie charts to be plotted on a monitor by, for example, translating figures produced by a database or spreadsheet or keyboard into a graph form. Dentists who are considering computerized tooth chartings would require graphics software to do so. The display of information in graphical form can be a great help in interpretation. Additionally, the monitor must be capable of utilizing the graphics software. It is important to ensure that the programs chosen are matched by the hardware on which they will run.

Databases

A database may be described as a computerized card index, or filing cabinet, with sophisticated retrieval and sorting capabilities. Records can contain information on whatever subject necessary, as well as names and addresses. Each record is divided into categories of information (known as 'fields'). The records can be laid out on the monitor in any format required and any one can be recalled instantly to be updated. Particular information from specific records can be used to compile selective mailings (known as 'mail-merge').

More importantly, database records can be used to produce reports on the information contained in the database. All dentists keep records of their patients, whatever their sphere of practice. Probably all record the name, address, telephone numbers, date of birth and sex of patients. Depending on individual preferences, other information may well be kept. In a database, one can create indexes for individual fields on which a search might be regularly conducted, to produce lists based on various selection criteria. A typical database record may include the following items:

- surname
- first name
- patient reference number
- date of last appointment
- recall date
- date of next hygienist appointment
- dentist code
- balance owed
- address
- home telephone number
- work telephone number
- date of birth
- sex
- full dentures (yes/no)

Of these items, for example, the surname, unique reference number, date of birth, dentist and denture references may be indexed.

One advantage of a computerized database is that the pattern of practice can be smoothed. For example, by means of patient reminders, a more even distribution of appointments can be achieved. Record misfiling can be minimized by leaving the computer to issue a unique reference number for every patient, which is then entered on the record card. As they are filed numerically, it becomes completely unnecessary to file record cards in strict alphabetical order, which can be difficult to achieve anyway. The computer can regularly generate an updated list of patients, in alphabetical order, with their numbers alongside, so that the cards may be retrieved easily. It is even possible to abandon record cards altogether, using a large complex hardware/software system.

The main core record of each individual patient, as described above, may be 'related' to several other databases used. This type of software package is known as a **relational database**. With these databases, the data held consists of several databases, or sets of files, with connections between them. These connections are specified by entering data into a field which is common to each file. For example, the patient's reference number (see above) is common to the main patient records, the payment and receipt transaction files, the laboratory work program and others. Whichever of the databases the staff are using, they will type in the patient's number and this will load from the main record the patient's name and any other required information. Relational databases can be set up quite simply, with little programming experience necessary, to be expanded later into complex and comprehensive management tools.

Many practitioners successfully restrict the use of their computers to peripheral purposes, unrelated directly to dentistry. Databases can be used very effectively for practice accounts, financial analysis and payroll.

Finally, a note of caution: there are a number of database programs available at a very modest price. However, they offer only limited facilities and, as the amount of information that most dentists need to store regarding their patients is so great, most practitioners would be disappointed with the results. One should consider spending any available money for software on a more comprehensive program.

Dental administration systems

Historically, dental administration systems have tended to be of two types:

- administrative systems, eg, recalls, payment receipts, simple practice accounting
- full clinical data systems, including chartings and treatment records

The administrative systems are much less costly, as they require less hard disk storage and simpler programs, depending upon the level of sophistication required. Conversely, the clinical types require larger storage capabilities, and more expensive hardware, with more advanced programming and faster processors.

Administrative systems

It is almost certain that every dentist would gain major benefits from the installation and use of a

[Patient Name]   [Current Date]
[Patient Address]

Dear [Patient Name]

Following an examination of the x-rays taken at your last visit, further treatment is indicated.

Would you kindly contact our receptionist as soon as possible to arrange an appointment. It would be helpful if you could advise her that your record card is filed in our 'letters sent' file.

Finally, please find enumerated below the amount of the charges payable for this additional treatment, together with the amount of charges outstanding, if any. Please pay for the amounts outstanding when you attend your appointment.

Yours sincerely

[Dentist Name]

PS.   We are only human and sometimes make mistakes! Thus, if you have made an appointment within the last couple of days, please ignore this letter.

Amount paid to date for this course of treatment: [X]
Balance payable for the treatment that you have already received: [Y]
The cost of your remaining treatment, if undertaken: [Z]

Figure 5.1

A sample computer-generated standard letter.

computerized dental administrative system. Patients' records carry vast amounts of valuable information. For example, using a central patients' database and a single machine, some of the following chores can be reduced to easily managed tasks:

- recalls
- referral letter writing
- incompleted treatment reminders
- telephone lists

- computerized appointment book and day-book listing
- payment information, analysis and automatic billing
- fee calculation
- laboratory checking and analysis.

In addition, simple practice accounting can be linked in, which might include payroll and automated stock control. For example, Figure 5.1 shows a computer-generated standard letter to a patient which, at the time of printing, automatically updates the patient's record to show the amount of the new balance owed.

There are now very many simple but valuable dental administrative systems available, starting from a modest price to expensive fully integrated all-purpose systems. It is worth spending some time in the practice to analyse the problem areas and then choose a system to solve the problem. The practitioner should not try to solve a problem that he does not have. For instance, there is no need to buy an appointment book program if the manual system is perfectly adequate.

Clinical systems

Abandoning the need for record cards and keeping all data in electronic records is a very attractive proposition for most dentists. There are already several very efficient systems available in most countries. They include beautiful chartings in graphic form and complex sort procedures to obtain data quickly from large storage mechanisms.

Before deciding to obtain this type of system, which by its nature requires powerful networking capabilities, with hardware in both clinical and administrative areas of the practice, several questions should be posed—with satisfactory answers given.

- Will the system be cost-effective, given the vastly increased costs involved?
- Will there still be a need for paper-based records for most of the patients, for the storage of X-rays, letters, estimates and other items?
- Will the practice still be able to function during power cuts, computer breakdown or periods of staff absence?
- Will staff training be any more difficult to accomplish properly, given the specialized nature of the program?

Purchase and maintenance

Hardware purchase

It has already been noted that the choice of hardware will depend mainly on what use the computer will have in the practice (see pages 53–4). The real beginner should not be persuaded by a suave salesman into the installation of a complicated networked multi-user system (which allows two or more people, using different terminals, to access the system at the same moment). A simple single-standing machine is the best way to start. This machine could probably be used later as part of a larger system, when proficiency has been gained and proper value judgements made.

Practitioners should consider carefully the relative merits of leasing or purchasing a computer. Recent history of hardware development indicates that hardware has become outdated within approximately five years. This does not mean that the computer becomes obsolete during this period, but software development is likely to be for newer machines after this time. The software would be designed to take advantage of any new features of the machines, so that purchasers of new software might be paying for features that they could not use.

If the purchase is for use in the practice, then having a fault repaired quickly could be quite crucial. It is preferable not to use mail-order for equipment purchase. This is fine for enthusiasts who know the insides of a machine—and thus how to change parts that go wrong—but beginners are likely to need professional help to install the machine properly, and fix any faults that occur soon afterwards.

Software purchase

Software is not actually bought—what is actually purchased is a licence to use it. Many packages are supplied with licence agreements that theoretically limit their use considerably. In practice, this does not cause any real difficulty.

Software is not likely to become obsolete as most major software packages are updated regularly, and registered users are given the opportunity to upgrade their packages to the newest version, at a modest cost. The newest version is normally indicated by a changed version number. For example, DOS started with version 1.1, went through versions 2.1, 3.0, 3.2, 3.3, 4.0 and so on. Applications software written for 4.0 may not work on the earlier versions—but conversely DOS 1.1 versions probably will work with all later ones.

There are several methods of obtaining software and, depending upon the complexity of the software, each might be used in different circumstances:

- 'bundled' with hardware
- from a specialized computer firm
- from a discount store
- from a user group

Many computers are now supplied with software included in the advertised price (known as 'bundled'). For some types of software, such as wordprocessing, this can be quite a good way of obtaining reasonable quality programs. There would be no harm in asking to try these programs as part of the decision to buy. However, it is important not to place too much reliance on such offers in the choice of either hardware or software. These programs tend to be either simple or outdated versions of well-known packages which can be obtained quite inexpensively anyway. The prices of some types of machines (especially those based on the old IBM-XT format) have become extremely competitive. It might be possible to persuade the dealer to give away some free software, in return for your order.

Obtaining software retail from a specialized computer firm is frequently—but not always—the method of choice. For instance, those purchasing specialist dental programs are likely to need much training and post-installation instruction. This will involve payment for the full price of the program and even for additional days of training and a software warranty with 'hot-line' support (where user queries are answered over the telephone). Conversely, for non-vocational programs, this may not be a good method of purchase. It is usual to find these being freely discounted in some of the computer magazines.

Purchased retail, from discount computer stores, most major packages are supplied with very good manuals of self-instruction for both installation and operation. A few hours of study and practice using the manual (and supplied tutorial disks) can help to make considerable financial savings.

User groups offer an excellent way of obtaining quite sophisticated software. Internationally, software developers have produced programs which have simply not been marketed through lack of resources. These programs have been placed in the 'public domain' either as public domain software, or as shareware (sometimes known as user-supported software). The former is truly free software. One joins a user-group for a modest annual subscription and then purchases disks of programs for about the cost of the disk itself. Usually, the program is complete with a manual which is on the disk itself and can be printed from disk onto paper. Shareware is obtained in a similar manner—the difference is that the user is honour-bound to register with the producer, after evaluating the software for a short period. The charge for this is very modest, and one obtains a complete version of the program, with extra functions, a bound manual, regular information and offers of updates. Wordprocessing, communications and other packages are available by this route.

However, it is important to ensure that only software from reputable clubs is obtained in this way, because of the danger of picking up a computer 'virus'. This is a program destruction code, usually written by an individual with extensive experience, which becomes embedded on part of a disk and is impossible to detect. The virus may be introduced by the programmer simply for vandalistic reasons. As the disk runs the virus attaches itself to programs and destroys them progressively by various means. While anti-virus programs are available, it is better to avoid viruses in the first place.

Maintenance

Computer hardware is normally very reliable, as it is electronically based. The incidence of breakdown reported is not high. The cost of having a computer repaired can be substantial – not only in terms of the expense of repair but also in terms of economic loss to the practice during the time of a fault, if much of the practice data or administration is computer-based. This is a typical computer-induced problem for any small business. To meet this problem, specialized hardware maintenance companies have evolved. The cost of this type of maintenance is based on 10 or 12.5 per cent of the full retail price of the hardware. The user may be guaranteed regular servicing of the equipment, attendances for repairs of breakdowns within two hours or so and no extra charge for the labour or parts replaced (whatever the age of the machine). Normally, the engineer will exchange the faulty part for a new or repaired one, rather than spending his time on site. In practice this type of agreement is essential.

Software maintenance is quite different. All the major well known programs are now 'bug-free' (free of faults) and do not require attention following their period of free warranty. Specialized programs, however, such as dental administration systems, tend to rely on the user to highlight faults, possibly months after installation. Some sort of extra warranty is thus essential. Maintenance agreements may often be obtained for a token extra charge at the time of purchase. It may entitle the user to 'hot-line' telephone support and updates to the main program as they are released. These warranties are usually well worth the money paid.

Making a start

There are three main elements to be considered when installing a computer in the practice:

● practice organization
● staff training
● after-sales maintenance and support

Practice organization

Practice organization is certainly the major element in the decision to computerize. There are several stages:

● Potential benefits to the practice should be identified, as well as existing difficulties. Software can then be selected to achieve these goals and to overcome the difficulties. Professional help from an independent consultant conversant with dentistry may be desirable.

● The appropriate equipment to operate this software should then be selected. It would be

sensible to ask colleagues' advice, in order to gain the benefit of their experience. For the novice, the plethora of hardware now being advertised can make the choice confusing.

● The administrative areas and operatories should be surveyed to establish whether there is room for the equipment, if it can be sited to fit in with existing power points, sterile areas and non-sterile furniture.

● If an all-embracing clinical system is chosen which dispenses with clinical notes, then decisions must be made on the storage and retrieval of record-card inserts such as conventional x-rays and referral letters.

● An installation plan should be drawn up. For example, this would include
– proposed date of installation
– arrangements for patients during installation
– possible operation of a parallel existing manual system during the settling-in and training period
– possible requirements for extra temporary staff to input data
It is necessary to decide whether to input existing data over a long period, as patients attend, or as one massive short-period exercise, using a rota of personnel working around the clock. The author's experience is that a short intensive period of data input is the most cost-effective and efficient method.

● Security of both hardware and software should be organized, to prevent theft or damage from fire or water. Data security should also protect against accidental or purposeful damage to data integrity. Staff should be issued with passwords that give access to appropriate levels of programs, depending upon their seniority within the organization.

Training staff

● Staff training can be formal or informal. Formal training may require the staff to devote their full time, for one or more days, to instruction in program techniques. Formal training is almost certainly essential for at least two members of staff, who can then carry out informal training for others.

● It is important to install software that is 'user-friendly' so that new and other members of staff can pick up the elements of the system with little formal training. 'User-friendly' means that programs and instructions are easy to understand with help easily available, preferably by on-screen information displays clearly labelled as such. Dentistry is a difficult enough vocation for the uninitiated to understand, without the added complication of complex software.

● On completion of training, specific tasks must be delegated to named personnel so that they can gain extra proficiency in the chosen area.

After-sales maintenance and support

● Maintenance is discussed on pages 63–4. It is important to be aware of what happens to the practice when something goes wrong—as it will.

● If the dentist installs a turnkey, all-embracing full clinical system, which dispenses with the need for record cards or written clinical notes, a decision will have to be made on how to operate when the system 'crashes' or if there is a power cut.

● Should it be impossible to continue in the event of some major breakdown, then obviously a rapid maintenance facility is essential—almost without regard to reasonable cost. An administrative-only system, however, may not require such an investment in rapid maintenance.

This chapter attempts to explain the advantages of computers in general dental practice and to encourage their increased use, as well as to introduce the basic terms and concepts. Practices with computers are thought of as modern and up-to-date by patients and their presence may assist in promoting a positive image, therefore encouraging the demand for dental care.

Glossary

application	Software designed for a specific task, eg, database.
ASCII	American Standard Code for Information Interchange: the codes of a keyboard which produce characters on a screen.
backup	Duplicate copy of software.
Baud	A unit of speed in communications programs.
byte	A unit of computer code, consisting of a group of adjacent binary digits (bits). Processors may work using 8-bits, 16-bits or 32-bits.
CGA	Colour Graphics Array: a colour screen which allows the display of graphics characters.
chip	A thin wafer made of silicone on which the electronic circuits are housed. Several will be arranged to form a CPU.
CPU	Central Processing Unit, also known as a microprocessor. See page 54.
database	A 'filing cabinet' of information upon which data processing can be performed to provide output.
disk drive	Holds floppy disk or hard disk and is usually built into the front of the CPU.
DTP	desktop publishing.
EGA	Enhanced Graphics Array: a screen which allows the display of sharp graphics characters, in mono.
floppy disk	A flat disk of magnetic-coated plastic enclosed in a plastic or cardboard case. It provides data storage, with a memory capacity of 360KB–1.4MB. Made in non-interchangeable sizes, 5.25 inches or 3.5 inches in diameter. It is removable from a disk drive.

FAT	On a disk, the file allocation table—the index which ensures that the disk can be read.
fonts	Printer typeface.
graphics	Any non-text information, such as graphs or cartoons.
hard disk	A sealed pack of internal special disks, spun continuously by an electric motor, which is located (usually permanently) within the casing that holds the CPU. May be anything from 20MB–300MB, much faster than floppy disks.
input	Data which is entered into the CPU.
kilobyte (KB)	Approximately 1000 bytes of memory (actually 1024 bytes), where one byte approximates to one letter, character or space of text.
megabyte (MB)	Approximately 1,000,000 bytes of memory (actually 1,048,576 bytes).
MHz	Megaherz; unit of speed of the CPU. May be 4.77–33 MHz.
modem	Device to control/convert ASCII code into a form that can be transmitted, often by telephone (origin: modulate/demodulate). The signal levels, speed of transmission and reception are measured in Baud. International standards may be 300–9600 Baud (30–960 characters per second).
mono(chrome)	Description of screen display when it is white or one colour letters on a black background, or blue/black letters on a white background.
MS-DOS	Microsoft Disk Operating System.
mouse	An alternative to the keyboard for controlling the movement of the cursor (pointer) across the screen.
multi-tasking	Describes a computer that is running several different programs simultaneously.
multi-user	Describes a computer or program capable of being accessed by several different users on different terminals at the same moment.
network	Two or more computers or peripheral devices, such as printers, which are joined by cable and which can exchange data.
output	Information produced by the CPU.
RAM	Random access memory: the part of the computer 'brain' in which the program is temporarily stored when it is in use. Usually 640K, or more. A program will not run if it requires RAM in excess of the computer RAM. See also page 55.
ROM	Read-only memory: usually not available for use by applications programs. It is not transient and so is not 'lost' when the computer is switched off. See also page 55.
spreadsheet	An application program which performs calculations on tables, rows and columns of figures.
turnkey	A term for a computer supplied with hardware and software purchased together, as fully integrated unit.
VDU	Visual display unit: the screen (UK).
VDT	Video display terminal: the screen (USA).
VGA	Video graphics array: a description of an extra sharp definition screen.
virus	A small piece of computer code that can automatically hide copies of itself inside legitimate programs. When a certain 'trigger' condition occurs, the virus may destroy valuable data and software.
WP	Wordprocessing: applications to create, edit, store and output text.

Part II   Team dentistry

6 Working in the seated posture

The increasing complexity of modern dentistry requires the dentist to perform greater amounts of work needing precise and accurate digital control and fine tolerances. In addition he has to maintain high levels of concentration for long periods of time. The effect is to increase tension and stress, both physical and mental (emotional), and there is no doubt that the practice of dentistry is extremely stressful (Fédération Dentaire International, 1985).

It seems that the image of dentistry as 'stressful profession' is an accepted part of dental culture (O'Shea, Corah and Ayers, 1984). Indeed even undergraduate students report severe discomfort in their backs, associated with musculoskeletal pain. Like their colleagues working in general practice, almost all dental students seem to accept this pain as part and parcel of their profession (Turley, 1983). However, those dentists who organize their dental office efficiently, work in a correct posture, with adequate lighting, and utilize chairside assistants and other ancillary staff effectively will:

- Maintain good health.
- Work with comfort, ease and efficiency.
- Perform clinical dentistry with minimum stress.
- Enjoy a smooth, relaxed day with a steady work flow.
- Work with much greater accuracy to produce a higher standard of work, because a relaxed operator is a better operator.
- Improve job satisfaction both for themselves and for their staff, through greater involvement and therefore better performance.

Causes of stress

These can be broadly classified into two main groups—physical and mental.

Physical stress

This is caused by body distortions due to:

- Incorrect working posture
- Poor vision of the operating point
- Difficult access to the operating point

Incorrect working posture

It has already been pointed out that working in a distorted posture leads to musculoskeletal pain, physical stress and disability; it also leads to loss of fine finger control. It is obvious from observing dentists at work that few of them are aware of the distorted postures in which they operate or of the abnormal and damaging physical stresses to which they subject their bodies by working in these postures. As long ago as 1964, Powell and Smith showed that dentists spend most of their working time in positions of anterior–posterior flexion, rotated counter-clockwise or bent laterally to the right. In approximately 70 per cent of cases studied by Powell and Smith, all three were present at the same time, this occurring principally in restorative operations.

Musculoskeletal pain and disability is caused by distortions which produce abnormal movements and tensions in joints and their attendant muscles, placing strains on those joints and causing asymmetrical muscle contractions. Figures 6.1 to 6.4 show many of the distortions most frequently observed in dentists at work:

- Excessive twisting and
- Over-flexion of the neck (Figures 6.1 and 6.2).
- Overloading of the thoracic vertebrae and shoulders by excessive flexion (Figure 6.3). The thoracic vertebrae are designed to give mainly rotational movement to the spine.

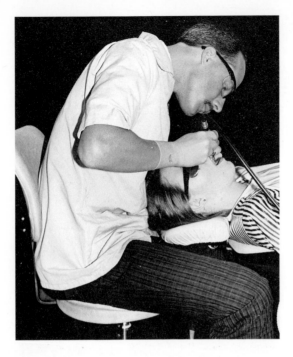

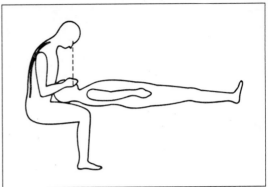

Figure 6.3

Over-flexion of the thoracic spine and flattening of the lumbar curve caused by the patient being placed too low down.

Figure 6.1

A dentist working on the left facial surfaces and showing: over-flexing and twisting of the thoracic and cervical spine; abduction of the right arm; raising of the right shoulder; over-splaying of the thighs.

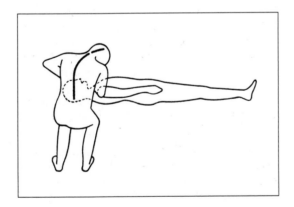

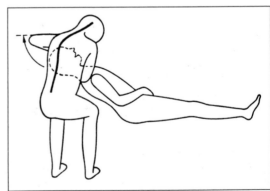

Figure 6.2

Bad working posture. Lateral torsion and over-flexion of the lumbar, thoracic and cervical spine caused by attempting to view the upper occlusal surfaces by direct instead of mirror vision.

Figure 6.4

Lateral torsion of the spine associated with excessive abduction of the left arm—caused by the patient not being fully supine.

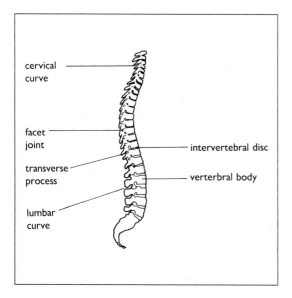

cervical curve

facet joint

transverse process

lumbar curve

intervertebral disc

verterbral body

Figure 6.5

The human spinal column showing lumbar and cervical curves, vertebral bodies, intervertebral discs, facet joints and transverse processes.

- Flattening of the lumbar curve (Figures 6.1 and 6.3).
- Excessive abduction of the thighs (because the chair backrest is placed between them) (see Figure 6.1).
- Excessive abduction of the upper arm and shoulder (Figure 6.4), which produces stress on the shoulder girdle.

It is the prolonged distortions which are damaging and produce permanent injury. For the standing operator, who is performing precision work at close focal distance, must be added the problems of fatigue and limb imbalance caused by placing all the body weight on one leg.

The problem is that most dentists are not aware of their working postures, nor of the presence of pain, because of the high level of their concentration on a small working point for a long period of time. Indeed most dentists accept musculoskeletal pain as a normal aspect of their working life and fail to realize how much this impairs their efficiency and the quality of their work. Dentists often only become aware of pain after they have finished working on the patient when their concentration has relaxed.

Many of the distortions described above can be eliminated by working at all times in the correct seated posture. In order to define this, it is helpful to consider briefly how the human spine functions.

The natural shape of the human spine is a shallow 'S' curve, with major concavities at the lumbar and cervical regions (Figure 6.5). Because of this 'S' shape, vertical load is absorbed in the same way as a coiled spring is compressed whereas, if the spinal column were a straight rod, vertical pressure would cause fracture. The vertebrae articulate with each other through joints at their articular processes known as facet joints. The individual vertebral bodies are separated from each other by the intervertebral discs. These help the vertebrae to move on each other to allow the spinal column to flex and they also act as shock absorbers to absorb vertical load.

Disc structure

The normal disc structure consists of:

- The annulus fibrosus, an outer ring of fibrous tissue, which has several layers. These are principally the circular fibres, which help to maintain the shape of the disc, and the oblique fibres, which pass between the vertebrae and help to limit rotation.
- The nucleus pulposus, an inner gelatinous layer, which acts as the hydraulic fluid of the spine. This constitutes the major part of the disc.

The discs are limited by the anterior and posterior longitudinal ligaments. It is the latter which is thinnest and in fact it is all that separates the disc from the spinal cord.

Back pain

Although a certain amount of disc degeneration (particularly of the annulus) takes place progressively throughout life, it is accelerated by abnormal

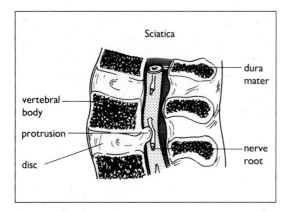

Figure 6.6

Compression of two vertebral bodies causing protrusion of the disc and pressure on the nerve root. In this example, in the lumbar spine, the prolapse would produce pain along the distribution of the sciatic nerve.

and asymmetrical pressures—very often caused by distorted posture. In such cases, excessive pressure is put on the nucleus, causing an intake of fluid and producing swelling; this in turn puts pressure on the annulus, and from thence onto the ligaments. The ligaments are innervated and so cause pain to be transmitted. Further breakdown of the annulus may result in prolapse of the disc content backwards (Figure 6.6), which will put pressure either on individual nerve roots, causing unilateral pain (for example sciatica), or directly on the spinal cord itself, causing bilateral pain (central disc prolapse).

With increasing age, pain may also originate from the adjoining facet joints, which become progressively osteo-arthritic. This situation is also aggravated by bad posture.

It would seem obvious therefore that, to prevent such lesions occurring, the dentist must work at all times in a correct and unstressed posture. Unfortunately there are several varying ideas about the true definition of correct seated posture. Many

of them are based on dogmas which have evolved without logical thought and show that few people have really examined this question properly.

Correct working posture

Posture may be defined as the relationship of jointed segments to each other. Because gravity acts on everything we do, the most natural and consistent movements and activities use gravity to our advantage. It is now generally accepted that a seated posture is the ideal one in which to perform fine, detailed finger activities requiring accuracy and thus close observation. The ideal seated posture will involve the smallest number of anti-gravity muscles.

In this ideal posture, there must be no abnormal bending, twisting or distortions in order to work. The preferred ideal posture must be maintained at all times and whatever the activity.

Where then does one begin to deduce logically what the correct working posture should be? This can best be done by means of a simple exercise. Observations by the author show that if any group of people is asked to sit in free space on a stool of correct height but without a backrest, and relax for 1 minute, it will be found that they all assume an identical posture in which:

- The long axis of the torso is vertical. The angle this axis makes with the long axis of the femur is known as the femur–trunk angle. Its importance will be described later in the chapter.
- The upper border of the thighs is at 15° to the horizontal.
- The upper arms hang vertically and loosely at the side of the torso.
- The elbows are in light contact with the side of the ribcage.
- The forearms are held loosely, below the horizontal, and the hands are clasped in the lap.
- The thighs are splayed by no more than 30° from the midsagittal plane.
- The head is erect, with the eyes looking straight ahead.

Such a posture is universal for all humans seated at rest and was first referred to by Dr Daryl Beach, of the Human Performance Institute, Atami, Japan, as the 'home position' (Beach, personal communication, 1974). It is from this posture that all

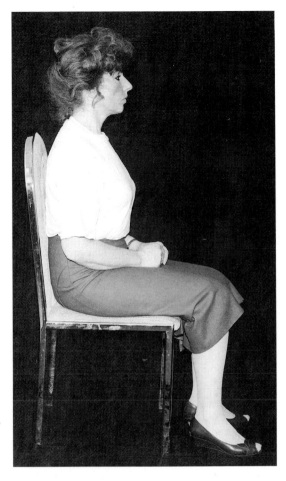

Figure 6.7

Subject seated in the resting ('home') position. The long axes of the torso and upper arm are vertical.

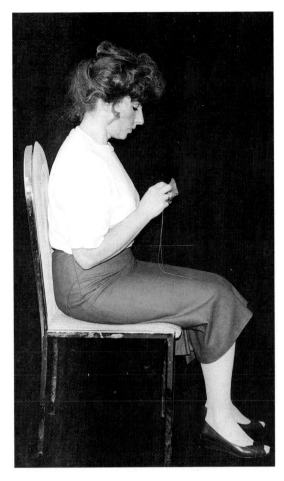

Figure 6.8

Subject seated and sewing a small piece of cloth. The forearms and hands are raised to mid-sternal height and the head is tilted for the eyes to observe the fingers.

organized human activity begins. Such a posture is totally relaxed and only the stabilizing muscles (those keeping the spinal column erect) are at work. None of the activity muscles (those needed to perform organized activity) are working.

If the same individuals are then asked to perform an activity such as writing, sewing (Figure 6.8), filing their nails, or gluing together small pieces of pottery—that is, a precision activity which uses the fingers and is closely observed by the eyes—these individuals will be seen to make only two movements:

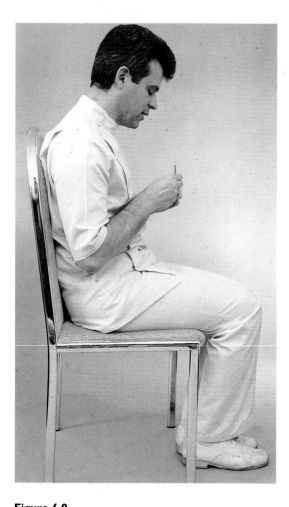

Figure 6.9

A dentist excavating a small cavity with the tooth held in space. The posture is identical to that shown in Figure 6.8.

● A raising of the forearms, pivoting at the elbow joint, so placing the fingertips at midsternal height and in the midsagittal plane.
● A forward tilt of the head so the eyes can observe the fingertips.

The only variation will be in the height from the ground at which the fingers are held and this is directly proportional to the degree of accuracy required for the particular task.

The same group are now asked to simulate operative dentistry. They are given a single tooth which has a cavity in it and asked to remove a small pencil dot from within that cavity using a very small excavator (Figure 6.9). This represents the working point. It is found that exactly the same two movements are made as for the other observed finger activities: that is, the tooth and the excavator are moved upwards to midsternal level and the head is tilted down for the eyes to observe the working tip of the excavator.

The height from the floor at which the tooth is held is determined purely by the height of the operator, as individual focal distance is subject only to minor variation. In all other respects, however, the posture of every member of the group will be identical, as the working point is held at midsternal level. Thus the ideal posture in which to perform operative dentistry has been logically deduced (performance logic). This may be defined as working with the highest degree of precision and control, with minimum of stress.

There is a further extremely important advantage of working in this posture. It has already been shown that it is the one naturally adopted when performing all closely observed tasks which require great precision and accuracy. This is because it produces maximum control, and therefore accuracy, of fine finger movements.

For this reason, the ideal working posture is referred to as the 'finger-control posture' (Figure 6.10), as described by Beach.

The finger-control posture

The criteria for the finger-control posture are as follows:

● The long axis of the torso is vertical. The maximum permitted tolerance is no more than 10° forward of the vertical.

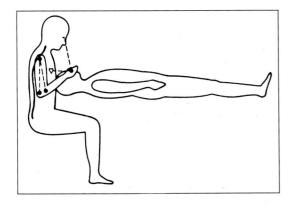

Figure 6.10

Criteria for the finger-control posture.

- The line of the shoulders is horizontal.
- The upper border of the thighs slopes at approximately 15° to the horizontal to produce the correct femur–trunk angle of 105° (see below).
- The thighs are splayed outwards no more than 30° to the midsagittal plane.
- The hip line is horizontal.
- The patient's mouth is in the midsagittal plane and the tooth at the dentist's midsternal level (Figure 6.9). This is the point midway between the superior and inferior sternal notches which is in fact approximately heart level.
- The upper arms hang vertically and the elbows are in contact with the side of the ribcage and not elevated or abducted.
- The forearms are elevated, pivoting at the elbow joint, placing the fingertips at the focal distance of the operator.
- The interpupillary axis is horizontal.
- The head is tilted forward no more than 30° to the vertical.

Such a posture will produce a balanced operator who has maximum control (and therefore accuracy) of his fingers. The muscles are centred and the total musculoskeletal system is in harmony and balance.

At this stage it is important to stress that the posture which has been defined so far is the one to be used for all precision work. In dentistry this is mostly confined to restorative and periodontal procedures. Many operative procedures which are performed beyond the dentist's focal distance can be done quite successfully with the patient seated upright and the dentist standing. Such procedures are usually those involved in prosthetics such as occlusal registration, shade selection, trying in and fitting of dentures, assessment of aesthetics for dentures, crowns, bridges and veneers, and face-bow registrations. Provided the dentist stands in a good upright posture, without distortion, there is nothing inherently stressful about the standing posture apart from physical fatigue if it is adopted for long periods of time. However, it is just as important to employ the 'five variables' (see pages 78–81) to ensure that the correct standing posture is maintained without stress. For example, when checking the shade and aesthetics of a full denture on a patient seated upright, the dentist should stand in the 7 o'clock location but should rotate the patient's head to the right so that the frontal plane of the face is parallel to that of the dentist.

The lumbar and cervical areas are perhaps the most common sites of pain for dentists and this is directly related to incorrect working posture. Close adherence to the principles defined for good posture will maintain the correct lumbar and cervical curves of the spinal column, eliminate abnormal pressures on the intervertebral discs, ligaments and nerves, and so reduce the possibility of producing the lesions referred to earlier in the chapter.

Seated height

It is important to clarify a common misconception about the correct seated height of the operator. For several decades, many writers and teachers have recommended, quite wrongly, that stool height should be such that the tops of the thighs

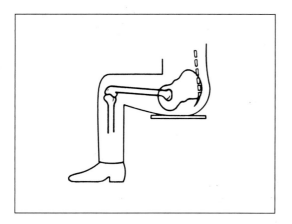

Figure 6.11

Sitting with the top of the thighs parallel to the ground produces a femur–trunk angle of 90° and causes flattening of the lumbar curve.

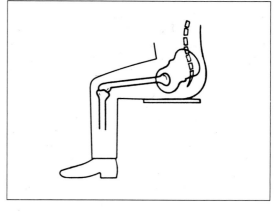

Figure 6.13

Sitting with the upper border of the thighs at 15° to the horizontal produces a correct femur–trunk angle of 105° and the correct lumbar curve is preserved.

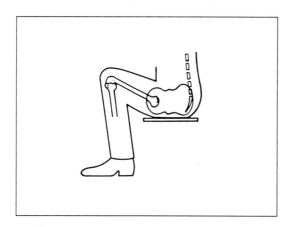

Figure 6.12

A femur–trunk angle of less than 90° produces even more severe flattening of the lumbar curve.

are parallel to the ground (Figure 6.11). Such a posture produces a femur–trunk angle of 90°. The effect of this is to reduce the lumbar curve, making it flatter (kyphosis). This causes the sacral and lumbar portions of the vertebral column to be pulled downwards, putting the lumbar spine under stress. As a result, the anterior borders of the lumbar vertebral bodies move closer together and cause pressure to be placed on the disc annulus, squeezing it backwards, with consequent pressure on individual nerve roots or directly on the spinal cord, as described earlier in the chapter.

Should the operator sit even lower than this, with a femur–trunk angle of less than 90° (Figure 6.12), as is common with many operators, then the lumbar curve is virtually eliminated, producing even more pressure on the discs by the vertebral bodies.

The original error arose because earlier researchers and writers overlooked the fact that the human thigh tapers from hip to knee and thus the definition of correct seated posture should have been based on having the *lower* border of the thigh parallel to the ground. This places the *upper* border at a 15° angle, producing a femur–trunk angle of 105° (Figure 6.13), which maintains the correct concavity of the lumbar curve and reduces pressure on the abdominal cavity.

The correct working posture has been defined by applying simple, logical analysis based on the principles of human engineering. Such a posture will enable the dentist to work not only with comfort and good health but with the greatest potential for fine finger control and consequently greater accuracy in his work.

The importance of good posture has hitherto been largely neglected in undergraduate training. The necessity for training students to work in the perfect posture was seen by Beach in the early 1970s. Many years of research and development resulted in the production of a clinical performance simulator, which was specifically designed to teach students at the beginning of their pre-clinical years to work in accordance with the principles of performance logic. The first such unit was installed in 1982 in the University of British Columbia and the second in the University of Maryland. The initial evaluation of the first year's experience was described in 1983 by Boyd and Donaldson.

Poor vision of, and difficult access to, the operating point

Both of these causes of physical stress can be eliminated by correctly utilizing a chairside DA and by applying the basic principles of chairside procedure. Both techniques are fully described in Parts II and III.

Mental stress

This is most commonly caused by:

- Lack of an efficient working system.
- Time pressures—incorrect use of the appointment book and poor management.
- Delays in the work sequence.
- Breaks in concentration.

The detailed causes of lack of efficiency and time pressures, and the solutions to these problems are fully described in Chapter 2, 3 and 4. Delays in the work sequence and the problem of loss of concentration are both caused by failure to apply the principles of work simplification or four-handed dentistry. The application of these techniques is fully described in Chapters 13 to 18.

7 Maintenance of correct posture

Having defined the correct working posture (the finger-control posture), it is important that it is maintained at all times, whatever the activity and whichever tooth surface is being treated. To permit the dentist to work in this way, the best position for the patient is fully supine. In fact, this is also the most relaxing position for the patient—being the natural rest position for all humans.

The 'parallel rule'

In order to ensure that the dentist is working in the correct posture for every clinical procedure, a simple guideline for him to follow is to maintain the frontal plane of his face parallel to the surface of the tooth being treated (Figure 7.1). This is the *parallel rule*. It ensures that the tooth surface is so located that a line from the dentist's eyes to that surface (or its reflected image if mirror vision is used) is as near to the perpendicular as possible. Only in this way can the dentist work in the finger-control posture for every surface of every tooth.

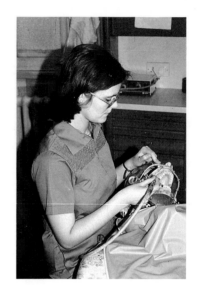

Figure 7.1

The 'parallel rule'. A dentist working with her frontal plane parallel to the right facial (buccal) surfaces.

The 'five variables'

To enable the dentist to keep to this very important parallel rule, there are five movement variations which he must incorporate into his working system. They are referred to as the *five variables* (Figure 7.2). These are:

- Location change by the dentist.
- Vertical height of the patient's mouth from the floor.
- Rotation of the patient's head left to right.
- Tilt of the patient's head forwards or backwards.

- Degree of opening or closure of the patient's mouth.

Location change by the dentist

Changes in operator location in relation to the patient's mouth are necessary for the dentist to adhere to the parallel rule. A seated operator on a mobile stool can move between the 12.30 and

78

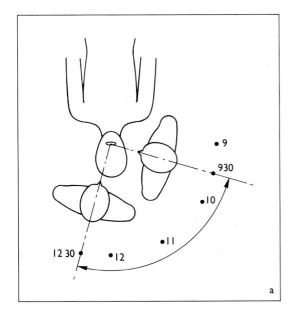

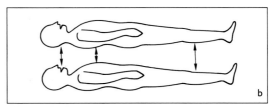

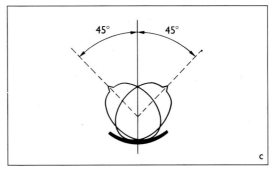

Figure 7.2

The 'five variables', showing: (a) location change, (b) vertical height change, (c) head rotation, (d) head tilt, (e) mouth open/closed.

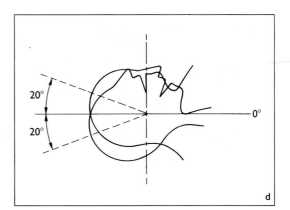

9.30 locations (Figure 7.2a). This range of movement is limited by the position of the DA seated to his left and by the patient's shoulder to his right. Movement past the 9.30 location would necessitate the dentist raising his right shoulder and arm in order to overcome the width of the patient's shoulders. This not only would place strain on the shoulder joint but also would result in twisting of the neck and excessive twisting and flexion of the thoracic spine (Figure 7.3).

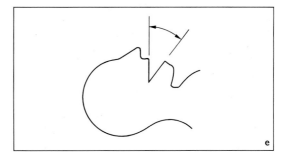

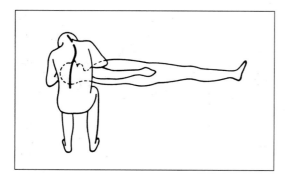

Figure 7.3

The probable shape of the spine of a dentist working beyond the 9.30 location. There is also lateral torque of the thoracic and cervical spine, because the right shoulder and arm are raised.

Similarly, movement further round than 12.30 would necessitate the DA moving away from the chairside and prevent her from gaining access to the mouth.

Vertical height of the patient from the floor

Vertical height of the patient from the floor can be varied by vertical movement of the dental chair (Figure 7.2b). This allows for variation in the focal (eye-to-tooth) distance of different operators. Thus the chair must be raised or lowered to the height at which the working point is at the dentist's close focal distance while maintaining finger-control posture. This is with the patient's mouth at midsternal height. Small variations in height must be made to compensate for changes in this distance, depending on the situation of the tooth in the arch. For example, the chair must be slightly higher for work on lower molars than it is for that on upper anteriors. This small movement, albeit no more than a few millimetres, must be made if the correct posture is to be maintained. Failure to be absolutely meticulous will produce a distorted working posture.

Rotation of the patient's head left to right

The limit of rotation is 45° either side of the vertical midline and this is well within the patient's comfort level (Figure 7.2c). For example if, when working on the facial surfaces of the right premolars, the patient's head were to be kept vertical and the dentist were to sit in the 12 o'clock location, the dentist would have to twist his neck and bend severely to his right to maintain the correct parallel relationship (Figure 7.4). If, however, the patient's head is rotated 45° to the left, the dentist is able to work in correct posture without distortion, since the facial surface is now brought parallel to his frontal plane and the eye-to-tooth line nearer to the vertical (Figure 7.5). This can sometimes be associated with a small change in location to 11 o'clock. In such cases, the amount of head rotation is less than for the 12 o'clock location.

Tilt of the patient's head forwards or backwards

A forward or backward tilt of the headrest (Figure 7.2d) permits changes in the inclination of the upper and lower occlusal planes to maintain the eye-to-tooth line as near perpendicular as possible. In general, most of the mandibular tooth surfaces can be seen by direct vision and the headrest should be tilted forwards. The amount of tilt depends on the individual patient's curve of Spee. For maxillary teeth beyond the cuspids, mirror vision is usually required and to facilitate vision the patient's head should be tilted as far back as possible. A maximum of 20° below the horizontal is usually found to be the limit of comfort for the patient. Any degree of tilt beyond this would cause strain on his neck.

Degree of opening or closure of the patient's mouth

With the patient's mouth opened wide, the tension of the cheek and the masseter muscles makes access difficult in the posterior quadrants. To provide greater access and better visibility, particularly in the posterior region, it is necessary to close the patient's mouth slightly, so relaxing the musculature and allowing the buccal soft tissue to be

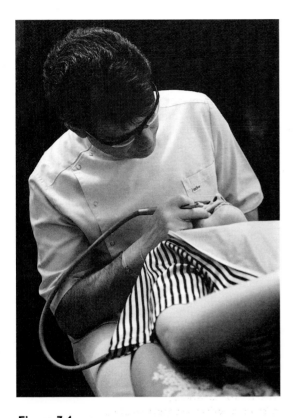

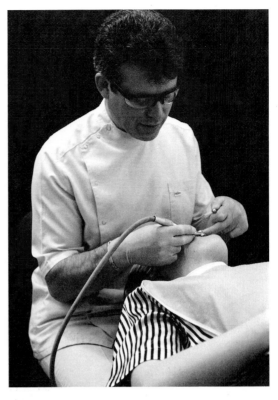

Figure 7.4

The dentist working in a distorted posture by attempting to view the upper facial (buccal) surfaces by direct vision from the 12 o'clock location.

Figure 7.5

The dentist in the correct finger-control posture looking directly down on the right facial (buccal) surfaces.

retracted. The maximum closure is approximately a two-finger width, which is the minimum opening required for placement of the aspirator tube and handpiece (Figure 7.2e).

Common faults in seated posture

For greater clarity, all the illustrations show the dentist at the 12 o'clock location. It must be emphasized that the following faults could occur in all the locations.

Fault

The dental chair is too low (Figure 7.6). This is the commonest fault among dentists who work

seated. It places the patient's mouth too far away so that, in order for the dentist to obtain an eye-to-mouth distance which is equal to his own focal length, he has to bring his eyes nearer to the patient's mouth by bending over. This causes over-flexion of his entire back and elimination of his lumbar curve. The effect of this is to alter the normal relationship of the vertebral bodies to each other, causing apposition of their anterior borders. This puts abnormal pressure on the discs, causing them to be squeezed distally and sometimes resulting in prolapse of the disc contents, as described on pages 71–2. Too low a position of the dental chair also produces excessive abduction of the thighs, since the headrest comes

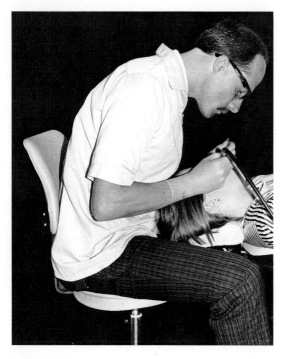

Figure 7.6

Faulty posture caused by to the patient's support being placed too low. This has caused the dentist to over-flex his thoracic and cervical vertebrae and eliminate the lumbar curve.

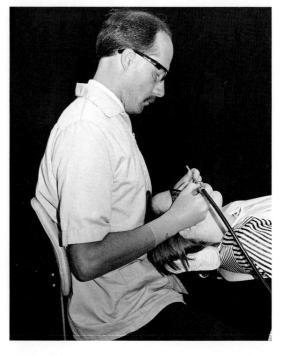

Figure 7.7

The dentist is working in the correct posture having raised the patient's support to place the mouth at mid-sternal level.

between them. This also forces the spine and pelvis forwards.

A further disadvantage is that it prevents the dentist making any location changes, since he is effectively locked in the 12 o'clock location by the presence of the chair back. The chances of obtaining the necessary parallel relationship are then greatly reduced and the likelihood of working in a distorted posture is increased.

Solution

The chair must be raised vertically to the correct height for the working point to be at the dentist's focal distance while he is in the finger-control posture (Figure 7.7). This restores the correct lumbar curve and in turn the correct relationship of vertebral bodies and discs. It also allows free movement to change locations because there is

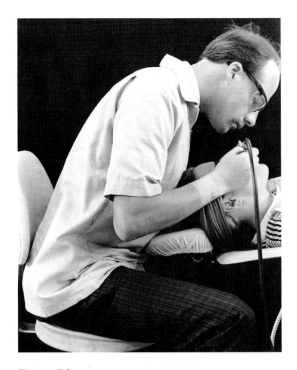

Figure 7.8

The patient's head is not at the top of the headrest and thus the dentist has to bend forwards.

In either case, for the dentist to maintain the vertical eye-to-tooth relationship necessary for good posture, he has to bend his back and neck excessively, which results in elimination of the lumbar curve and over-flexion of the thoracic and cervical vertebrae. The further away from the top of the headrest the patient's head is placed, the greater the degree of over-flexion and distortion by the dentist.

Solution

The solution is for the DA to ask the patient to move up towards the top end of the chair, to the point where the top of the patient's head is level with the top edge of the headrest (see Figure 8.8). This is a most important duty and must be meticulously carried out before the dentist begins work on the patient. The dentist should then move in towards the chair until he is virtually in contact with the patient's shoulder when working in the 10 or 11 o'clock location or the top of the patient's head when working in the 12 o'clock location. The closer to the patient the dentist works, the better will be his working posture. When changing location, the dentist will tend to lose this close contact with the patient because he moves in the arc of a circle. Any change of location must therefore be accompanied by a slight inwards movement towards the patient, to restore close contact.

space between the dentist's thighs and the back of the chair.

Fault

The dentist works too far away from the chair. The patient's head is not at the extreme end of the head-rest (Figure 7.8).

Fault

The chair back is not totally horizontal so that the long axis of the patient's torso is at an angle greater than zero (Figure 7.9). This will also result in excessive flexion of the dentist's neck and back and elimination of his lumbar curve if he is to obtain the necessary eye-to-tooth line. In addition, it will cause the dentist to raise and abduct both his shoulders and upper arms and will produce severe strain in these areas. The further forward the

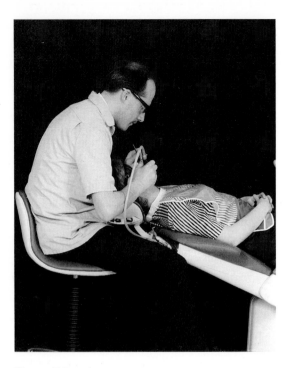

Figure 7.9

The chair back and headrest are not horizontal. The dentist is leaning forward causing over-flexion of his spine and he has abducted his thighs because he cannot place his legs beneath the chair.

backrest is tilted from the horizontal, the greater the degree of bending by the dentist.

Personal observation shows this to be one of the commonest faults in dentists' working posture, largely because it is the mistaken belief of many dentists that patients are unwilling or unable to lie totally supine.

There are two reasons for this totally misguided attitude: concern about patient resistance and fear that the supine patient is likely to gag.

Patient resistance

Many dentists believe that patients will find the fully supine position unnatural and uncomfortable, and will resist it. This is in fact a totally fallacious view. Provided patients are in normal health and the correct technique for seating them is followed (see pages 92–3), they find it natural and comfortable to lie totally flat. After all this is the same position as they adopt when sleeping in bed. It is only when there is deviation from the horizontal, such as the head being lower than the torso or the legs elevated, that the patient feels insecure and uncomfortable.

Gagging

Some dentists fear that the supine patient will gag from accumulation of water in the mouth. However, the fully supine patient is far less likely to gag than the one lying on a chair with the backrest raised. Schön (1972) has clearly demonstrated that, if the patient is fully horizontal, the soft palate and dorsum of the tongue close together, and seal off the pharynx. This seal is opened as the patient is raised. In addition the gag reflex is depressed in the fully horizontal posture. For these reasons, the more horizontally placed is the patient, the less likely he is to gag, while the further forward the backrest is raised, the more likely the patient is to gag.

Solution

The solution is to lower the backrest as flat as possible (see Figure 8.1) so that the patient's torso is horizontal. This is fully discussed on pages 92–3.

Fault

The backrest is horizontal but the headrest is tilted too far forwards. This causes similar distortions to those just described.

Solution

The solution is to adjust the headrest in accordance with the principles of the five variables (see Figure 7.2). Other than when working on mandibular teeth by direct vision, the frontal plane of the patient's face should never be above the horizontal. In those dental chairs in which the backrest cannot go completely horizontal, this can be compensated for by tilting the headrest further back. Conversely a dental chair which has the capability of being lowered to the totally horizontal requires less backward tilt of the headrest to maintain the frontal plane of the patient's face horizontal.

Fault

Excessive twisting of the dentist's cervical and thoracic vertebrae (see Figures 6.1 and 7.4). This is caused by the dentist attempting to view facial surfaces of premolar and molar teeth by direct vision without employing any of the five variables.

Solution

The solution is for the dentist to change location and rotate the patient's head.

Fault

Lateral flexion and horizontal rotation of the thoracic spine beyond normal limits (see Figures 6.1 and 6.4). These distortions tend to occur together. The major causes are usually:

- Viewing by direct vision without employing the five variables.
- The chair backrest raised above the horizontal.
- The headrest raised too far above the horizontal.

- Using direct vision for surfaces which should only be viewed by mirror vision.

Solution

The solution is to maintain the patient fully supine and to use the appropriate variables—usually rotation of the patient's head—and to use mirror vision where necessary (see pages 110–15).

The operating stool

The need to work in the ideal posture has been emphasized. An operating stool designed to allow the dentist to do this must thus be regarded as a most important necessity. An ideal stool would have the following features:

- A rectangular, comfortably padded seat with the right degree of firmness to provide support.
- A seat area wide enough to give full buttock support and long enough to support at least two-thirds of the length of the thigh.
- A leading edge which is curved slightly downwards to provide a 'waterfall effect' so that the vessels of the thigh are not compressed.
- A backrest which is firm, non-flexible and, most importantly, shaped convexly, with sufficient curvature to give positive support to the lumbar curve.
- A wide base with five castors making it easily mobile to facilitate location changes.
- An easy seat-height adjustment. This can be either manual or gas lift.

There are very many designs of operating stools which do not possess these features (Figure 7.10). Among the most common faults are a round seat of insufficient area giving no support for the buttocks and thighs; a flexible backrest which does not give any lumbar support; a hard leading edge with no 'waterfall', causing compression of blood vessels; and a difficult height-adjustment system.

Some authorities maintain that an ideal stool should incorporate the additional feature of a seat which tilts as the operator bends forward. This is

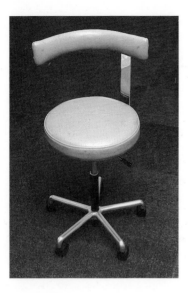

Figure 7.10

An unsuitable design of dental stool with a round seat of inadequate area and no lumbar support.

based on the work of Mandal (1976), who noted that people who perform finger activity slouch forwards instead of sitting upright. Stools with a seat tilt are said to necessitate less flexion at the hip joint in order to keep the torso vertical and to re-establish the lumbar curve. However, careful adherence to the criteria for achieving good posture as described in this chapter make this an unnecessary luxury. In addition, it has the disadvantage of reducing the operator stability which is so necessary for accurate finger control.

The role of magnifying loupes

Magnifying loupes are optical systems which provide the dentist with a magnified image of the patient's mouth and teeth together with a wide field of view. They are extremely effective in reducing working stress and, at the same time, they improve accuracy of work (Paul, 1988). The most basic types are simple magnifying lens which either clip onto the dentist's spectacles or are retained by a headband. However, these have the disadvantage of requiring the dentist to tilt his head downwards in order to focus on the operating point. This leads to over-flexion of the cervical vertebrae and so contributes to physical distortion and stress.

By far the best type is that known as telescopic. Telescopic loupes incorporate special prisms which 'bend' the incoming light rays so that the dentist does not need to over-flex his neck to obtain vision. There is a range of magnification levels currently available but the most commonly used are 2.5× and 4× magnification. This type of loupe is fitted to the dentist's own spectacles (either plain or prescription) using a lightweight inter-pupillary distance bar clipped onto the frame and can be flipped upwards out of the way when not required. It must be stressed that telescopic loupes have to be individually fitted by the manufacturer, with great accuracy, paying special attention to the correct inter-pupillary distance for each dentist. If desired, telescopic loupes can be fitted with a miniature spotlight which focuses on the working point and gives a small, concentrated beam of high intensity. Some dentists employ this means of illumination as an alternative to a fibre-optic light fitted to the handpieces. Certainly both these types of high-intensity illumination are particularly advantageous in improving visual acuity and so contribute to a higher degree of accuracy as well as maintenance of a good working posture. The choice of which method to use is very much a personal one.

Advantages

- *Diagnosis*: Small lesions not visible to the naked eye are often observed.
- *Treatment*: Cavity and crown margins can be finished more smoothly and with a higher degree of accuracy.
- *Restorations*: The placing and polishing of restorations, particularly of composite resins, are greatly improved using magnification.
- *Crown and bridge procedures*: The marginal fit can be seen far more accurately.

● *Working posture*: Improved working posture is often an unrecognized advantage of using loupes. Any attempt to over-flex the neck or spine by bending over the patient to see more clearly is prevented because the image seen through the loupe will not remain in focus unless the correct focal distance is meticulously adhered to. This therefore causes the dentist to sit in a more upright, and therefore less stressful, posture.

Once the dentist becomes accustomed to working with loupes, he rarely returns to practising without them. It is necessary to explain to the patient exactly what the loupes are and why the dentist wears them, but patient reaction is almost invariably favourable. After all, it clearly conveys to the patient the fact that the dentist is working to a very high level of accuracy, an obvious benefit to the patient.

Exercise

As with any sedentary occupation, it is essential to take regular exercise. Swimming is perhaps the ideal one for dentists and DAs, since it has a beneficial effect on the spine and entire musculo-skeletal system. The water supports the body so that a full range of exercise is possible without placing strain on joints and muscles. During the working day, it is important to stretch and walk around the office between patients and, also occasionally, during prolonged operative procedures.

Stretching, clasping the hands behind the back, arching the spine, breathing deeply and flexing the fingers are all useful exercises which should be performed frequently if the dentist is sitting for long periods.

8 Efficient utilization of the dental assistant

For the dentist to be able to work with maximum efficiency and in the correct posture, the utilization of a skilled chairside assistant—the well-known 'four-handed' or 'close-support' technique, also termed dental auxiliary utilization (DAU)—is essential.

The aim of the technique is to delegate as many non-operative tasks as is ethically permissible to a well-trained DA who works at the chairside with the dentist for the whole of the time he is treating the patient (Figure 8.1). The two must work together as a dental team.

Four-handed dentistry is an essential part of good practice management in that it reduces stress and increases productivity. There are still many dentists who fail to realize this and continue to employ one assistant who acts as both receptionist and DA. The two jobs require totally different skills and temperaments, and such a situation usually results in neither of them being done satisfactorily. It also precludes the possibility of the dentist having the full-time benefit of a chairside assistant which is so fundamental to team dentistry. For this reason, *two* people must be employed, one dealing with reception and the other with dental assisting duties. There is, of course, no reason why each should not be also trained in the basic skills of the other's work, so that they can cover in cases of short-term absence.

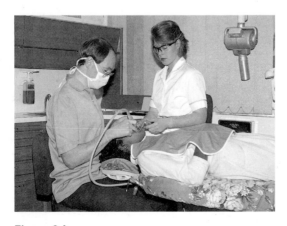

Figure 8.1

A dentist and DA correctly seated to form a chairside team. The patient is totally horizontal.

Advantages of the four-handed technique

- Reduction in stress and fatigue for the dentist.
- Improved vision of the operating point.
- Improved finger control and accuracy.
- A higher standard of dental care.
- Increased working efficiency.
- Maximum use of the dentist's chairside time.
- A more relaxed working day.
- An increase in the DA's work potential.
- Greater job satisfaction for the DA. This can in turn often act as a catalyst to the enthusiasm of the dentist.
- Improved dentist–patient relationship.
- A more relaxed patient. The presence of a kind and sympathetic assistant gives reassurance to

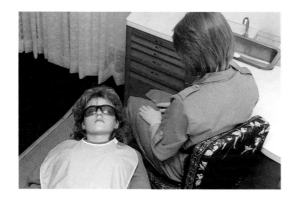

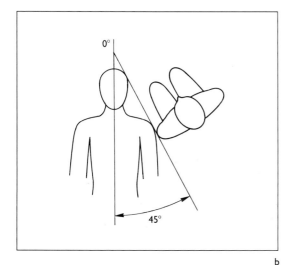

b

Figure 8.2

Correct location of the DA, seated with left hip opposite the patient's shoulder (a) and with thighs at 45° to the long axis of the patient (b). This locates the DA as close to the oral cavity as is physically possible, without bending her back.

the patient and helps to reduce his apprehension (Paul, 1971).

The dentist must never take for granted the work done by the DA or fail to appreciate her value in improving the quality of his working life.

Correct seated position of the dental assistant

Ideally the DA must be seated comfortably, stably, with a good posture and with a clear and uninterrupted view of the operating field.

- Her posture must be as near as possible to that of the dentist. However, it must be remembered that the DA's work does not involve such close observation as that of the dentist so she does not need to work within her close focal distance. Unlike the dentist, most of her work involves hand and arm, not finger, movement. For this reason, her eye to mouth distance can be greater than that of the dentist—indeed it must be so if she is sitting in the correct position.
- Because the DA is seated at a fixed distance from the patient's mouth (Figure 8.2), any forward movement of her hands should be achieved by extending her arms forwards towards the mouth. In this way, the DA can maintain her torso vertical and retain the lumbar curve. If she were to try to work at her close focal distance with her elbows in contact with her ribs, she would need to bend forward and across the patient's body, with consequent overflexion of her back, causing stress and back pain.
- Her location should be at 3.30 relative to the patient (Figure 8.1).
- Her left hip should be level with, and as near as possible, to the patient's upper arm, at a point almost opposite the patient's shoulder (Figure 8.2a). For the taller DA, this point may come as far as half-way towards the patient's elbow.
- The long axis of her thighs should be approximately parallel to a line between the tip of the patient's left shoulder and left ear. This line is at about 45° to the long axis of the patient (Figure 8.2b).
- Her seated height should be such that her eye level is 10 cm higher than that of the dentist

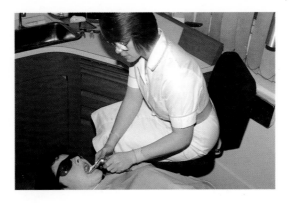

Figure 8.3

The DA is seated too far down the chair away from the patient's shoulder, producing severe distortion and over-flexion of her back.

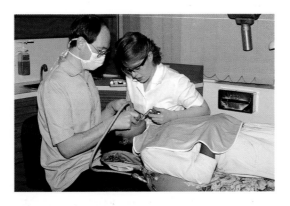

Figure 8.4

The DA is seated too low and has to bend over in order to gain a view of the mouth.

(Figure 8.1) because she must be able to see over his hands to obtain proper vision of the mouth. Such a seated height is necessary because the DA is seated slightly further away from the patient's mouth than is the dentist.

● A line from her eye to the patient's mouth should be as near vertical as is possible. The greater the angle between this line and the horizontal plane, the better the view of the mouth. However, because the DA is further away from the mouth than is the dentist, it is rarely possible for this angle to be greater than about 60°.

● The DA should be able to rotate her stool without twisting at the hip and waist to gain access to her work surfaces and materials.

Common faults in the assistant's seated position

Seated too far down the dental chair

A common fault is for the DA to be seated too far down the dental chair towards the footrest so that her hip is level with the patient's elbow or forearm. To obtain vision of the mouth from this position requires severe bending of the back (Figure 8.3). Moving further upwards towards the headrest corrects this by placing the DA's left hip level with the patient's upper arm (Figure 8.2).

Seated too low

This causes the DA to flex her back because she has to arch forwards to obtain vision of the mouth (Figure 8.4). In addition, she has to raise and abduct her arms and shoulders to overcome the obstruction of the patient's body. This produces severe stress in the shoulder joints and muscles.

Incorrect angle

If the DA is seated so that the long axis of her thighs is at a right angle to the long axis of the

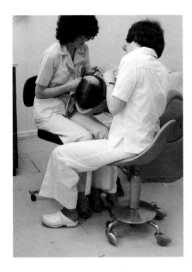

Figure 8.5

The dentist and DA seated at 9 o'clock and 3 o'clock, facing each other. The dentist is working in a severely distorted posture with a lateral tilt of both her back and neck. The DA's back is over-flexed.

patient's body, she is placed further away from the mouth, because the distance from the hip joint to the knee joint is greater than the distances between the two hip joints. This position produces a severe over-flexion of her back in order to obtain vision.

Incorrect location

Another common seating error is for the DA to be seated at a 3 o'clock location, with the dentist seated at 9 o'clock, and the DA's legs placed between those of the dentist (Figure 8.5). There are many disadvantages of this position:

- It locks both the DA and the dentist into a fixed position and eliminates the possibility of either of them changing location.
- It causes the dentist to sit with thighs splayed and excessively abducted—a distorted working posture.
- It increases the distance from the DA's eyes to the patient's mouth, and causes her to over-flex her spine to achieve vision of the mouth (see above).

The ideal stool for the dental assistant

Like the dentist, the DA must be seated comfortably if she is to work effectively and without stress. She must therefore have a suitable stool with the following features:

- A frame which will place the seat higher than that of the dentist.
- A broad footrest on which she may place her feet since she will be seated higher.
- A seat of shape and area similar to that required for the dentist's stool (see page 85).
- A seat which rotates easily, so that the DA can move from the working point in the mouth to her work surface by rotating the seat instead of twisting her body.
- Glides instead of castors, to provide greater stability.

A mobile stool is not required and indeed would be a distinct disadvantage. The DA does *not* need to change location and her duties, in particular aspiration and mixing of materials, demand that she works from a firm and stable base.

Duties of the dental assistant

- Prepares and organizes the treatment area.
- Seats the patient correctly.
- Prepares the patient for treatment.
- Maintains a clear operating field.
- Assists with the control of soft tissues and maintains access for the dentist.

- Maintains clear vision of the operating point within the tooth.
- Prepares materials.
- Passes and exchanges hand instruments.
- Anticipates the needs of the dentist.

These duties will be considered in detail in the remainder of this chapter and in Chapters 9–11.

Preparation of the treatment area

- To prevent cross-infection, all work surfaces must be wiped down with one of the many suitable disinfecting solutions available. These are most easily applied from a spray bottle, but impregnated wipes are also available which are activated on being dampened. All air turbines, motors and air–water syringe tips should be removed, autoclaved and replaced by sterilized ones. It is therefore necessary to have duplicates of all of these items. Sterilization and disinfection procedures are fully described in Chapter 12.
- All record cards for the day must be checked against the day list and placed in the treatment room in correct order.
- A check must be made that all laboratory work required for the day has been returned, as described in Chapter 3.
- The appropriate treatment tray and materials required must be laid out.

Seating the patient

It has to be accepted that all patients are apprehensive. Many, particularly the older ones, also express a dislike of being in the supine position in the dental chair. This is largely because the dentist employs an incorrect method of placing the patient in the horizontal position.

Most dentists seat the patient in an upright chair and then slowly lower the backrest to the horizontal position. It is this very motion of the backrest which produces a feeling of insecurity, disquiet and apprehension in the patient rather than the supine position itself. A further disadvantage is that in most cases the movement of the backrest to the

Correct seating of the patient

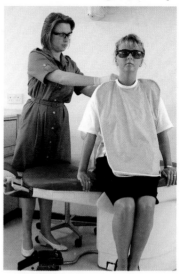

Figure 8.6

When the previous patient has left the treatment area, the chair is left in the fully horizontal position. As the next patient enters, she is asked to sit on the chair edge and the DA puts the protective bib in place. Protective spectacles may be placed either before or after the patient is in position and either by the patient or the DA.

horizontal causes the patient's head to move away from the top of the headrest. This will produce a distorted work posture for the dentist from excessive flexion of the spine as described in Chapter 6. The DA must always ask the patient to move up to the top end of the chair to a point such that the top of the patient's head is coincident with the top of the headrest (see Figure 8.8). This is a most important duty and must be meticulously carried out before the dentist begins working on the patient.

There is a better method of seating the patient which virtually eliminates the patient's resistance to the supine position. The chair must be set horizontally before the patient takes up position. The patient is then actively guided into the correct supine position by the DA (see Figures 8.6–8.8).

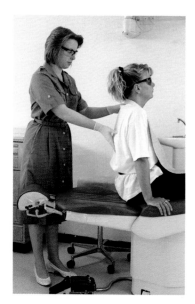

Figure 8.7

The DA then puts her right hand behind the patient's back, in contact with the shoulders, and asks the patient to lie down. The physical presence of her hand on the patient's back is reassuring and comforting and removes the feeling of insecurity and apprehension. The DA maintains this hand contact until just before the patient is totally supine.

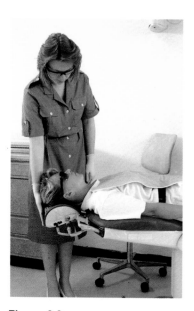

Figure 8.8

Finally the DA checks that the top of the patient's head is level with the end of the headrest.

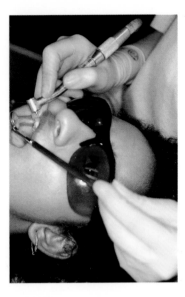

Figure 8.9

Curved protective spectacles do not interfere with the placement of the dentist's left hand.

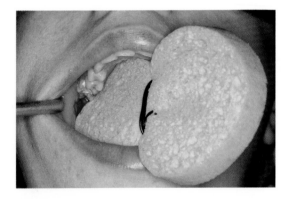

Figure 8.10

A protective sponge placed in the mouth extends back into the fauces area and gives access to the entire upper right quadrant.

It has been found that patients prefer this method of seating because it removes much of the disquiet associated with the backward movement of the backrest. It virtually eliminates any objection or patient resistance to the use of the supine position. An additional advantage is that it is more likely to ensure that the patient's head is at the top of the headrest than the first method.

At the end of treatment the reverse procedure is applied. The helping hand of the DA can again be placed behind the patient's shoulders to give positive support whilst he sits up.

This technique is also particularly good for young children, who find it quite natural to climb onto the flat chair and with the DA's help to lie down with their head in the correct position.

Although it is normally essential for the patient to be totally horizontal, there are a few exceptions to this rule. These include patients in advanced pregnancy, and those with hypertension, bronchitis, emphysema, hiatus hernia and with spinal ankylosis. In the last case, the aim should be to try to place the patient's head so that the frontal plane is horizontal. It is helpful to place a cushion under the shoulders for the patient's comfort. In such a case it is necessary for the dentist to raise the height of his stool, since the height of the dental chair is raised. It must be emphasized that, provided health reasons do not preclude them lying flat, all patients, at whatever age, can lie totally horizontal without discomfort. Indeed, because this posture is physically relaxing for patients, it also helps them to feel more mentally relaxed and therefore less apprehensive.

Preparation of the patient for treatment

Eye protection

The use of high-speed rotary-cutting instruments, high-pressure air syringes and acid etchant materials, coupled with the use of hand instruments in close proximity to the patient's mouth, makes it essential for eye protection to be provided, not only for the dentist and the assistant but also for the patient.

Protective spectacles for the dentist and the DA can be of any type, either in glass or plastic, provided they are comfortable and give adequate eye coverage. Those provided for the patient, however, must fulfil special criteria. They must be curved convexly in both directions so that there is total protection by precluding the possibility of debris going beneath the edges. An additional advantage of this design is that the convex curve of the spectacle frame prevents the corners obtruding into the dentist's work area and interfering with normal placement of his hands, and so allows him to maintain a natural operating position (Figure 8.9). The sharp, upstanding corners of conventional spectacles would provide a mechanical obstruction to correct hand position. In addition there is a danger that the dentist's hand may catch the side of such spectacles and either knock them off or traumatize the patient.

For these reasons, the DA should always remove the patient's own spectacles, if worn, and replace them with the correct curved ones. These may also be tinted, which helps to relax many patients and cuts out a great deal of glare from the operating light. This factor has become increasingly important with the advent of high-intensity light-curing units.

Protecting the patient's airway

Though it has been shown that the oral vestibule of the totally supine patient is mechanically closed off by the apposition of the soft palate and tongue (Schön, 1972), there is still the danger that small objects may drop down past this barrier and either be swallowed or pass into the airway. To avoid this danger, either a tightly packed, cotton-filled gauze pack or, preferably, a butterfly sponge pack, should be placed in the mouth to protect the airway. This acts as a mechanical barrier and must be used in all situations involving the trial, removal and cementing of temporary and permanent crowns, inlays, bridges, veneers, posts, pins and small prostheses. The DA must therefore always prepare a sponge or gauze pack and be ready to hand it to the dentist before any of these types of treatment commences. The sponge is preferred because it is denser than a gauze pack and less likely to allow heavy objects (such as metal bridges or crowns) to displace it. The DA should first dampen the sponge and then hand it to the dentist, who will place it into position, just distal to the tooth being treated (Figure 8.10). The dentist must ensure that the pack is spread across the entire oral cavity, though it should *not* be packed deeply into the patient's throat, but merely used as a mechanical barrier.

9 Maintenance of a clear operating field

The removal of coolant water and saliva from the oral cavity is an essential duty of the DA in order to maintain a clear working field for the dentist and also for the patient's comfort. The process is variously referred to as aspiration, high-volume evacuation or, more simply, suction. All these terms refer to high-velocity, high-volume aspiration of fluid. For the sake of simplicity, the terms 'aspiration' and 'aspirator' will be used throughout.

Aspiration

Ideally aspirators should have:

- The capability of operating with a low pressure.
- An on/off switch which cuts in and out automatically when the aspirator tube is removed and replaced.
- A filter for solids which is easily cleanable.
- No unduly sharp bends in the pipes in which debris will be deposited.

The suction motor should be powerful enough to remove fluid at the rate of $10.28\,m^3/min$, with a 10 mm diameter of tube under a negative pressure of 127 mm. Central suction systems are preferable to the mobile variety, since they are less space-consuming and more hygienic, with no reservoir bottle to empty. However, the importance of checking and cleaning all aspirator tubes and systems very frequently and replacing filters regularly cannot be over-emphasized. After every patient, the system should be cleaned thoroughly by aspirating clear water containing a suitable cleanser. Fluids are now available which also incorporate a disinfectant.

Design of the aspirator tube

Ideally this must be:

- Of large enough diameter to evacuate fluids at the required rate.
- Bevelled at the tip to provide maximum area for suction.
- Capable of being held by the DA in a comfortable palm grip without strain on her wrist or fingers.
- Shaped so that, when in use, the DA's hand does not obscure her own view of the mouth.
- Easily rotatable to change the relation of the bevel to the tooth.
- Non-traumatic to the patient's soft tissues.
- Disposable or autoclavable up to 134°C/273.2°F.

The basic types of aspirator tube are: straight (Figure 9.1A), slightly curved (Figure 9.1B) and obtuse angled (Figure 9.1C).

Straight and curved tubes

Straight and slightly curved aspirator tubes are basically similar and will be considered together here. Tubes of this type are usually 6 or 9 mm in diameter and are made of metal or plastic. Some are bevelled at one end to about 45°.

To obtain maximum suction area, the bevel should be held parallel to the tooth being prepared. To achieve this, there are two basic grips used to hold the straight and curved designs of tube.

Pen grip

The tube is held as if holding a pen, with the thumb and first two fingers in the long axis pointing

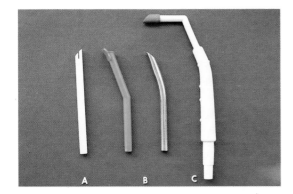

Figure 9.1

Different designs of aspirator tubes: (A) straight, (B) curved and (C) obtuse angled.

towards the mouth (Figure 9.2). This places great strain on the DA's wrist and fingers, particularly on the extensor tendons. The strain is increased considerably if the patient has strong oral or tongue muscles and the control of these tissues can be extremely difficult in such cases.

Reverse palm–thumb grip

The tube is held using all four fingers and with the thumb extending backwards along the tube, pointing towards the DA's body (Figure 9.3). This gives a firmer and more controlled grip but produces an even more unbalanced and strained position of the DA's wrist, forearm and indeed the complete shoulder girdle. The strain is also accentuated if the patient has strong oral muscles. It is not recommended as a usable grip.

Disadvantages of straight and curved tubes

- Both grips block the DA's view of the mouth (Figure 9.4). This causes her to lean sideways, usually to the left, in order to obtain vision, so placing her in a very distorted and stressful posture.
- To maintain the bevel parallel necessitates the DA holding her hand too high, which not only obscures her view of the mouth but often interferes with the dentist's correct hand position (see Figure 9.2).
- To maintain the bevel parallel necessitates rotating the entire tube in the holder.
- The sharp end of the tube, whether plastic or metal, can traumatize the patient's tissues.

Obtuse-angled tubes

These are placed in a palm-grip type of holder. This type of design fulfils most of the ideal criteria for an aspirator tube.

- The special holder is of correct shape and size to be held in a comfortable palm grip (Figure 9.5). This eliminates strain on the DA's fingers, wrist and arm.
- The correct angle between holder and tube permits the DA's hand to be so placed that it does not obscure her view of the mouth (Figure 9.6). This allows her to sit in an unstrained posture.
- The design places the DA's hand outside the dentist's work area. This eliminates the interference with the correct placement of his hand (Figure 9.7).
- The vinyl tip is soft and non-traumatic to the patient's tissues.
- The tip is separate from the tube and can be easily rotated to change the relation of the bevel without rotating the entire tube.
- Tissue retraction is easier and less traumatic for the patient because of the mechanical advantage of the angled design, which requires less pressure for retraction of soft tissues.
- It incorporates a built-in crosspiece, which acts as a filter for large pieces of solid debris and eliminates the possibility of blockage of the system.

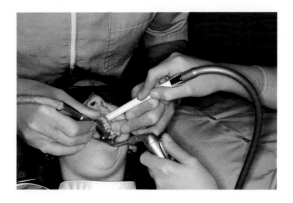

Figure 9.2

A straight tube held in a pen grasp. There is strain on the DA's fingers and obtrusion into the dentist's working area.

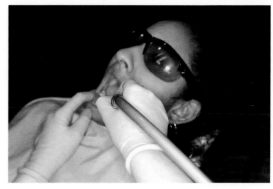

Figure 9.4

The DA's view of the mouth is blocked when holding a straight or curved aspirator tube.

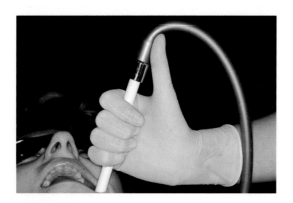

Figure 9.3

Reverse palm–thumb grasp. There is severe strain on the DA's fingers and wrist.

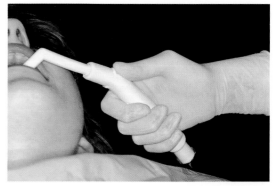

Figure 9.5

The obtuse-angled aspirator tube held in a comfortable palm grip with no finger or wrist strain.

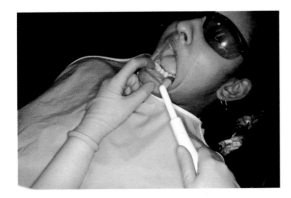

Figure 9.6

When holding an obtuse-angled aspirator tube, the DA has a clear and unobstructed view of the mouth.

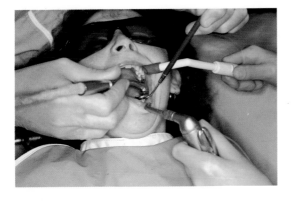

Figure 9.7

The obtuse-angled aspirator tube held in a palm grip does not interfere with placement of the dentist's hand.

There are two such designs currently available, integrated and adaptable. Both systems can be autoclaved up to 134 °C/273.2 °F.

Integrated high-volume evacuator

The integrated system is made of metal, with the holder as a self-retracting integral component of the chair unit. Only the obtuse-angled tube and vinyl tip are removable for sterilization. Because the holder is fixed into the chair, it is non-removable and cannot be used with any other aspirator systems.

Adaptable system

The adaptable system consists of a palm-grip holder and obtuse-angle tube, which *can* be removed from the vacuum hose. It is available in an inexpensive kit form. It incorporates a multi-diameter adaptor which fits all known models of aspirator tubing, making it truly universal (see Figure 9.1C).

Principles of aspiration

To ensure maximum evacuation of fluid, the provision of an unobscured view for the dentist and the avoidance of trauma to the patient's soft tissues, it is mandatory that:

- The aspirator tube or holder must always be held in the DA's right hand (see Figures 9.2–9.7). Her left hand must always be free to retract soft tissues, exchange instruments, hold the three-in-one syringe and wipe the working end of instruments while they are still held by the dentist.
- The tip of the tube should always be on that side of the dental arch nearest to the DA (see Figures 9.2–9.7).
- The DA's hand and the aspirator tube must never obtrude into the dentist's work area.
- For this reason, when the dentist is working on the lower left quadrant, the DA must not retract the tongue by placing the aspirator tube lingually. Were she to do so, her hand and the tube would completely block the dentist's view,

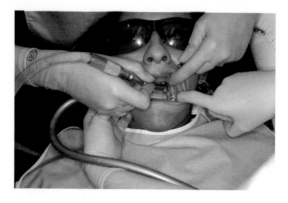

Figure 9.8

Aspiration of the lower left quadrant by holding the aspirator tube on the lingual side. There is strain on the DA's wrist and interference with the dentist's hand position.

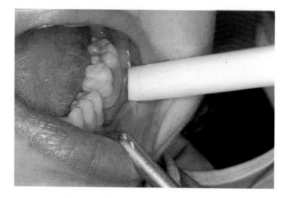

Figure 9.9

On-site placement of the tip for aspiration of the lower left quadrant.

interfere with the correct placement of his working hand (Figure 9.8) and force him to move into a distorted working posture in order to see the operating point.

● The tip must never touch the soft palate or go beyond the anterior pillar of the fauces as this will induce the patient's gag reflex.

Intra-oral positions of the aspirator tube

There are two basic positions:

● *On Site*: This must be used when the tube is required to retract soft tissues.
● *In the Fauces*: This can be used when the tube is not required to retract soft tissues.

On-site position

● The tip is sited adjacent to the tooth being prepared (Figure 9.9).
● Its bevel is parallel to the buccal or lingual surface of that tooth. This provides the maximum surface area and therefore evacuates the maximum volume of fluid. There is one exception to this rule. When operating on the lower right quadrant, the tongue and/or sub-lingual tissues are often drawn into the opening of the tube, causing it to be blocked. This can be prevented by the DA rotating the tube through 90° (Figure 9.10). This places the longest portion of the tip on top of the tongue, which can then be gently depressed, and prevents the tongue from blocking the orifice (Figure 9.11). The small loss of evacuation efficiency is more than compensated for by eliminating the tube blockage.
● The top of the tube must be level with the occlusal surface of the tooth. It must never be held higher than this because it would interfere with the dentist's access to the tooth.
● The bevel should be not less than 1 cm away from the tooth to avoid diversion of the coolant spray from the bur head.

Careful attention to these principles will ensure that water is drawn across the tooth during preparation, thus maximizing the cooling effect.

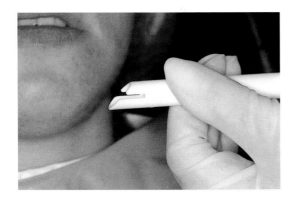

Figure 9.10

Rotation of the tube through 90° prior to aspirating the lower right quadrant.

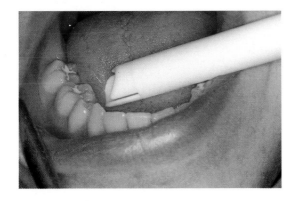

Figure 9.11

Aspiration of the lower right quadrant—the aspirator tip bevel has been rotated and depresses the tongue.

Fauces position

The tip is placed approximately 3 mm lingual to the pterygomandibular raphe, just lingual and distal to the last molar tooth (Figure 9.12). Because all coolant water and saliva collects in the fauces when the patient is supine, it is the ideal position for the aspirator tip, provided it is not required for retraction of soft tissues. An additional advantage is that the tip is completely away from the dentist's intra-oral working area.

Occasionally, on-site suction does not remove all water and fluids. In such cases, any accumulation of fluid in the fauces can be removed by a combination of the two techniques. The DA moves the tip from the on-site position to the fauces position, picks up the water, and moves the tip back on site with a quick movement of her wrist. It must be emphasized that this must not be done while the bur is revolving, since the loss of retraction provided by the on-site position may allow the soft tissue to fall onto the rotating bur, resulting in trauma.

The fauces position is also used during high-speed cutting of the right maxillary molars and of the anterior teeth.

High-speed cutting of left maxillary molars

There is insufficient space between the cheek and the maxillary molar teeth for both aspirator tip and handpiece. If positioned on site, the aspirator tip would prevent placement of the handpiece head and the dentist's finger-rest (Figure 9.13). In this situation, the tip should be placed in the fauces position of the opposite (contralateral) side instead of on-site (Figure 9.14). This will provide adequate evacuation of fluids while still allowing the dentist access to this area.

Additional space can also be obtained by asking the patient to translate his mandible to the left and so opening up the buccal space. Almost all patients can perform the movement with ease.

High-speed cutting of anterior teeth

Though technically the aspirator should be on site to retract the lip, its placement in this position does not remove sufficient water, so the fauces position is preferred. However, in this situation, the water

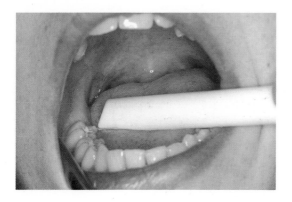

Figure 9.12

The fauces position of the aspirator tip just distal to the last molar tooth.

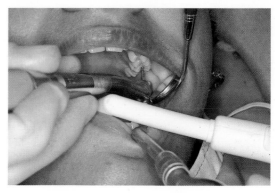

Figure 9.14

When working on the upper left molar area, the aspirator tip is moved across into the contralateral fauces position.

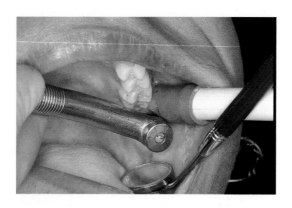

Figure 9.13

On-site position of the tip for the upper left molars, showing occlusion of space for the dentist's handpiece.

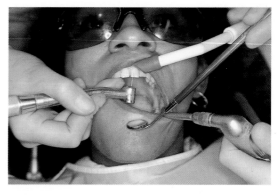

Figure 9.15

Retraction of the upper lip using the aspirator tip—the bevel has been rotated through 90°. Two cotton rolls placed in the upper labial sulcus retract the lip both upwards and away from the gingival margin.

spray usually impinges on the patient's face and into the nostrils, causing some discomfort and often inhibiting nasal breathing. To avoid this situation, two cotton-wool rolls should be placed in the labial sulci, one on either side of the frenum. This has the

dual effect of both retracting and everting the upper lip, which gives the dentist better vision and also forms a mechanical barrier between the spray and the patient's face.

Additional and more positive retraction should

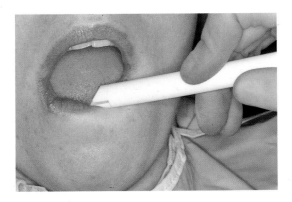

Figure 9.16

The tip has been incorrectly inserted into the mouth, trapping the lower lip and causing trauma.

Table 9.1 Aspirator tip positions.

Upper left quadrant	Adjacent to the facial (buccal) surfaces of the teeth (Figure 9.9)
Lower left quadrant	
Upper right quadrant	Fauces position (Figure 9.12)
Lower right quadrant	Adjacent to the lingual surfaces of the teeth (bevel rotated through 90°) (Figure 9.11)
Maxillary anteriors	Fauces position for high-speed cutting
Mandibular anteriors	On-site position (bevel rotated), if retraction is required (Figure 9.15)

be provided by the middle finger of the dentist's right hand. Since direct vision is being used, the mirror can be rotated back into his palm, so freeing the middle finger for use in retraction (see page 106 and Figure 10.1).

Since the tube is now not required for lip retraction, it can be placed in the fauces position.

However, when the dentist views the palatal surfaces of anterior teeth, he has to use mirror vision, so he can no longer use his right third finger to retract the lip. Though the labially placed cotton rolls are usually sufficient to retract the lip, additional retraction by the DA using the aspirator tip (Figure 9.15) or syringe is extremely helpful because it provides better vision and illumination of the palatal surfaces.

When the dentist uses the slow-speed handpiece for preparation on the palatal surface, because of the absence of spray the aspirator tip can be always placed on site. This provides more positive retraction and allows the DA to use her air–water syringe to wash and dry the cavity and mirror.

In this situation the bevel of the aspirator must be rotated through 90° upwards for upper teeth (Figure 9.15) and downwards for lower teeth to retract the lips while preventing them blocking the opening of the tube.

A summary of aspirator-tip positions is given in Table 9.1.

Correct insertion of the aspirator tip

- When inserting the tip, the DA must be careful not to traumatize the patient's lip (Figure 9.16).
- The DA must place the aspirator tip in position intra-orally before the dentist places any instrument in the mouth.

This last point will ensure that the tip is precisely placed in the correct position to the advantage of both dentist and DA. Almost invariably it is found that the dentist places his handpiece and mirror into the mouth before the DA inserts the aspirator tip. The effect of this is to leave insufficient room and makes it very difficult for the DA to gain proper access. She is forced to fit her aspirator tip into whatever available space remains and is accordingly unable to place it correctly. In these circumstances, the DA must ask the dentist to remove his mirror and handpiece from the mouth, to allow her to place the aspirator tip correctly.

To avoid trauma and ensure the aspirator tip is correctly placed, there are two ways in which it may be inserted, using either the finger or the tip of the air-water syringe to gain access (Figures 9.17–9.21).

Method I

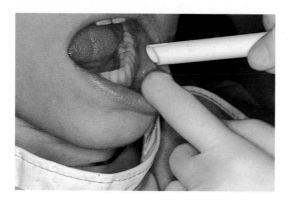

Figure 9.17

The DA gently pulls back the lip from the dental arch using her left index finger.

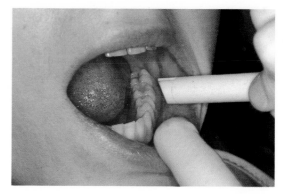

Figure 9.19

The tip is angulated through 30° and moved outward into the buccal sulcus to the on-site position. This will retract both the cheek and the lip. Secondary retraction of the lip is maintained by keeping the index finger in position. This technique not only provides greater safety but also prevents the lip blocking the light source and gives better illumination of the operating point for the dentist.

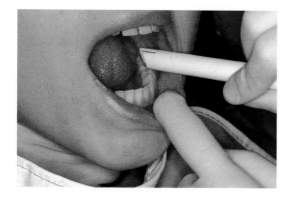

Figure 9.18

The tip of the aspirator may then be inserted, slid distally along the arch to the molar region.

Method 2

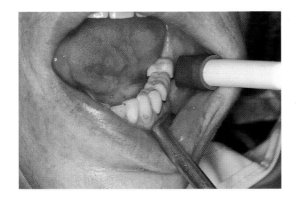

Figure 9.20

If an air–water syringe is availabe on the DA's side, it is preferable to use this to pull back the lip and for use for secondary retraction. In order not to traumatize the gingivae, the side of the syringe tip should be used. The advantage of this method is that the syringe is available for washing and drying of the operating site.

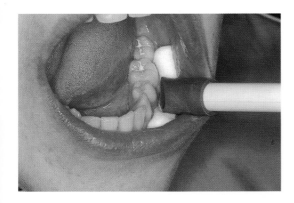

Figure 9.21

Access can be further improved if necessary by placing a cotton roll in the sulcus before placing the aspirator, which can then be rested on the roll. Either of these methods must be used whether the vacuum tip is placed buccally or lingually to the teeth.

Ideally both the dentist and the DA should have their own air-water syringes. If, however, only one is available, it must be transferred to the DA's side because she will use it more frequently than the dentist.

This can usually be facilitated with minimal expense by fitting a longer air line which allows sufficient length to be run under the chair back and for the syringe to be placed in a holder which is fixed to the side of the DA's work surface.

10 Maintenance of operating vision

Soft-tissue control

Control of the patient's lips, cheeks and tongue is essential:

- To protect the integrity of these tissues. This is particularly important with the use of high-speed rotary-cutting instruments, which can so easily traumatize them.
- To maintain access to, and vision of, the operating site for the dentist.

Soft-tissue retraction must be carried out according to the following rules:

- Retraction of those tissues on the side of the arch facing the dentist is the responsibility of the dentist.
- Retraction of those tissues on the side of the arch facing the DA is the responsibility of the DA.

Soft tissue may be retracted by means of the following:

- The dentist's finger-rest (preferably his middle finger).
- The DA's left index finger.
- The tip of the aspirator.
- The tip of the air–water syringe.

Any one of these methods for primary retraction can be supplemented by any of the others for secondary (subsidiary) retraction.

Techniques of retraction

Lower left cheek and lip

Primary retraction: aspirator tip.
Secondary retraction: DA's index finger or air–water syringe tip.

These methods of retraction are fully described in Chapter 9 and shown in Figures 9.17 to 9.21.

Upper left cheek and lip

Primary retraction: aspirator tip.
Secondary retraction: dentist's left middle finger.

These methods of retraction are the same as described for the lower left except that the aspirator tip is placed on site at the upper arch and no secondary retraction is used by the DA. Should such retraction be necessary, it is better for the dentist to provide this by using the middle finger of his left hand (Figure 10.1). He should not use the front surface of his mouth mirror for the retraction (Figure 10.2) because of its tendency to slip off the moist surface of the mucosa, with the consequent possibility of trauma to the lip.

The other disadvantage of using the mirror for retraction is that it places greater strain on the fingers, wrist and shoulder because the longer distance necessitates the elbow and upper arm being abducted from the side of the body. Using the left middle finger provides not only more firm and positive retraction but also eliminates this stress by allowing the dentist to maintain his elbow in contact with the side of his body. Because of its greater length, it is preferable to use the middle finger rather than the index one.

Lower right cheek and lip

Primary retraction: dentist.
Secondary retraction: DA.

These tissues are retracted by the dentist using his right middle finger as a finger-rest for the hand-piece (Figure 10.3). This will automatically retract

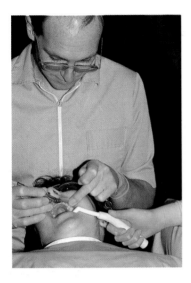

Figure 10.1

The dentist retracting the upper left lip and cheek using the middle finger of his left hand. His upper arm is vertical and his elbow correctly in contact with the side of his body.

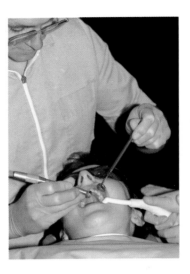

Figure 10.2

Incorrect method of retraction of the upper left lip and cheek using a mouth mirror. The mirror tends to slip off the mucosa. Note also that the dentist's torso is tilted to the right and his upper arm and elbow are abducted away from the side of his body.

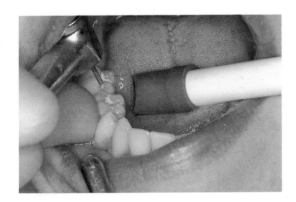

Figure 10.3

Retraction of the lower right lip by the dentist's finger-rest with accessory retraction from the DA's air–water syringe.

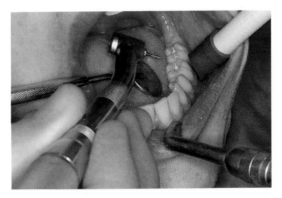

Figure 10.4

Incorrect method of retraction of the tongue on the lower left by using a mouth mirror.

the cheek and lips. If necessary, secondary retraction may be provided by the DA using the air–water syringe tip or her left index finger to retract the lip and give improved illumination to the quadrant. The aspirator tip is maintained on site on the lingual side of the arch to retract and protect the tongue.

Upper right cheek and lip

> Primary retraction: dentist.
> Secondary retraction: DA.

The method is the same as that described for the lower right. However, the aspirator tip is here placed in the fauces position since there is no requirement to retract soft tissue.

Tongue—Lower left

> Primary retraction: dentist's mirror.
> Secondary retraction: none.

It is often wrongly assumed that the best way to retract the tongue away from the lower left arch is to pull it towards the midline using either the front of the dental mirror (Figure 10.4) or a flanged saliva ejector. However, this is a most unnatural action for the tongue since the natural movement of its musculature is in a vertical not a horizontal plane. This technique therefore tends to cause the tongue to react against the retracting source, which compounds rather than helps the problem. In addition both of these instruments, particularly the flanged saliva ejector, occlude the available space and prevent proper access for the dentist.

Correct method

The back of the dental mirror is used to depress the tongue vertically using the technique illustrated in Figures 10.5–10.8.

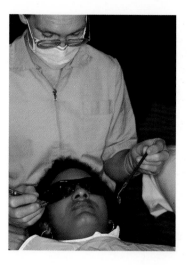

Correct method for retraction of the tongue: lower left

Figure 10.5

The dentist grasps the mouth mirror handle at its extreme end between the thumb and index finger, using the middle finger as a rest. This is the 'long mirror' grip referred to later in the chapter (see Figure 10.17). If the patient has a very active tongue, the fourth and fifth fingers may have to be utilised to exert slightly more pressure. The dentist rotates the mirror between his index finger and thumb, moving the mirror head through 180° from its normal viewing position so that its reflecting surface is pointing towards the DA.

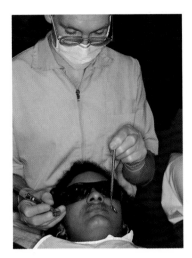

Figure 10.6

He moves his left forearm from left to right and inwards towards his chest. In effect this moves the mirror handle from left to right across the midline of the patient's face.

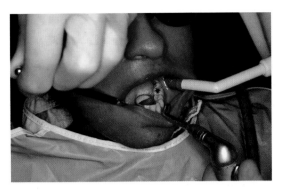

Figure 10.8

The dentist then places the under-surface of the mirror head on the tongue and depresses it vertically to a level about 1 mm below the gingival margin. In this way the tongue is moved vertically in its natural direction. There is no reflex counter-reaction from the patient because the contact is a very light one and so the tongue does not over-react against this force. This retraction technique should be used for all preparations in the left mandibular teeth.

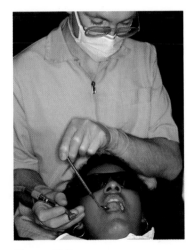

Figure 10.7

The dentist continues to move his forearm inwards and upwards, approximating his left hand to the right of the patient's face with his palm facing downwards until the mirror head is horizontal. This is a natural human movement since the shape of the elbow joint dictates that the forearm always moves upwards and inwards towards the midsagittal plane. It is precisely the same movement as that made when folding the arms.

The technique is not difficult to learn and with a little perseverance is easy to apply. It is both very comfortable and an effective operating position. The forearm and hand are totally supported by the dentist's chest and this allows him to control even the most difficult tongue without strain on his wrist or fingers. The technique is particularly useful for preparations involving molar lingual surfaces because the free access allows the handpiece to be placed horizontally across the mirror head (Figure 10.9).

Tongue—Lower right

Primary retraction: DA.
Secondary retraction: dentist's mirror.

The tongue is retracted by the DA using her aspirator tip placed on site adjacent to the lingual

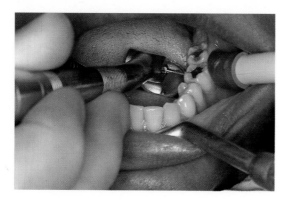

Figure 10.9

The handpiece head can be placed across a horizontal mirror when cutting lower left lingual surfaces.

Table 10.1 Soft-tissue retraction.

Tissue	Primary responsibility	Method of retraction
Upper and lower left cheeks	DA	Aspirator tip
Upper and lower left lips	DA	Left index finger or air–water syringe tip
Upper and lower right cheeks Upper and lower right lips	Dentist	Finger-rest of right hand
Upper and lower lips midline	Dentist	Middle finger of left hand
Left tongue	Dentist	Mouth mirror
Right tongue	DA	Aspirator tip (bevel rotated 90°)

surface of the tooth (see Figure 9.11). The bevel is rotated through 90° as previously described. Such a method of retraction automatically keeps the tongue below the level of the dental arch. Where the patient's tongue is difficult to control, extra retraction can be provided by the dentist using the back of his mirror.

Secondary retraction of the lower lip may be provided by the DA's left index finger or the tip of the air–water syringe, but this should always be placed anterior to the tooth being prepared in order not to obtrude into the dentist's working area (see Figure 9.11).

Upper and lower lips

The use of cotton-wool rolls to provide primary retraction in the anterior region has been referred to in Chapter 9. Though this is helpful in providing retraction, it has to be emphasized that positive, and therefore safe, retraction of the lips in the anterior region can *only* be achieved by the dentist carrying out the retraction with the middle finger of his left hand.

The responsibilities for retraction must be clearly demarcated and are summarized in Table 10.1.

Mirror vision

It must be accepted that, while the use of the five variables (see page 78) will enable the dentist to see a greater number of tooth surfaces by direct vision, there are still a number of surfaces for which reflected or mirror vision must be used, if correct working posture is to be maintained. When using mirror vision, the parallel principle described on pages 78–80 must be applied. The only difference is that the dentist maintains his frontal plane parallel to the mirror surface rather than to the tooth surface itself. To achieve and maintain this relationship to the mirror, the five variables described on pages 78–80 must be employed in precisely the same way as for direct vision. One of the principal reasons why many dentists try to avoid using mirror vision is because it becomes obscured either by back-spray from the high-speed handpiece during cutting or by debris deposited during later stages of cavity preparation. When the mirror is

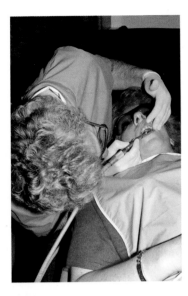

Figure 10.10

Dentist viewing the upper palatal surfaces by direct vision, causing him to work in a distorted posture.

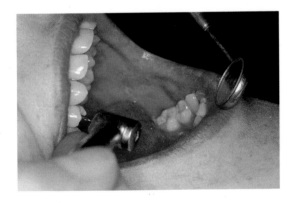

Figure 10.11

The dry-zone technique. The mirror is positioned in front of the high-speed handpiece.

held directly below the cavity, and therefore below the high-speed handpiece, fine spray droplets fall onto its surface and cloud the reflected image. Because his vision is therefore obscured, the dentist attempts to view the preparation by direct vision (Figure 10.10). Invariably this can only be achieved by distorting his working posture. The reflective properties of the mirror must therefore be maintained throughout the procedure by ensuring it is free of fine spray droplets. There are two methods of achieving this: prevention by use of the dry-zone technique and removal using a surfactant.

Prevention

Spray can be prevented from falling onto the mirror by using the dry-zone technique. Instead of holding the mirror beneath the tooth being prepared, the dentist places it in front of the turbine head by at least 1 cm (Figure 10.11). Spray droplets falling vertically therefore do not drop onto the mirror. To help obtain this relationship, the mirror head is placed level with the mandibular occlusal plane in one of four positions, producing four views:

- Mirror position 1
  The mirror head is placed at the lingual surface of the right mandibular cuspid (Figure 10.12).

- Mirror position 2
  The mirror head is placed level with the lingual surface of the right mandibular second molar.

- Mirror position 3
  The mirror head is maintained level with the buccal surface of the right mandibular second molar.

- Mirror position 4
  The mirror head is placed at the labial (facial) surface of the right mandibular incisors or cuspid (Figure 10.13). This position is variable and can be maintained anywhere from the red margin of the lip to the outside of the mouth depending on the angulation of the upper teeth.

All these mirror positions can be used for both left and right quadrants of the mouth. For viewing the upper left quadrant, the positions are identical but

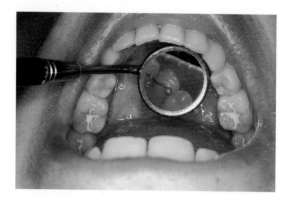

Figure 10.12

Mirror position I—adjacent to the lingual surface of the lower right cuspid.

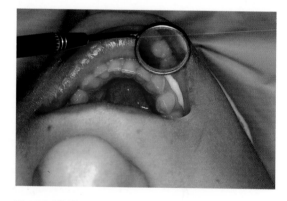

Figure 10.13

Mirror position 4—adjacent to the facial surface of the lower right cuspid.

the mirror is related to the left cuspid and molar. It will be found that in the majority of cases, only positions I and 4 will separate the mirror and the handpiece sufficiently to provide the necessary dry zone, and, in practice, in high-speed cutting these are the positions used almost exclusively.

Although in many cases this method will ensure that the mirror is not obscured by spray falling upon it, it has to be accepted that in some situations the technique is ineffective. This may be due to excessive volume of spray but is usually because spray is reflected in a random direction from both cuspal inclines and cavity angles. In such cases an additional method must be used.

Removal of spray from the mirror surface

The mirror surface should be coated with an agent which will reduce surface tension. This can be either a solution into which the mirror can be dipped or an aerosol spray which the DA can spray onto the mirror surface (Figure 10.14). If the solution is used, it must be changed for every patient to avoid cross-infection; the spray is preferable, being more hygienic.

The wetting agent present on the mirror will cause the fine droplets of spray to coalesce into a uniform, plane film of water. Although the mirror surface is wet, it will still give a perfect reflection (Figure 10.15). Wetting agent must be con-tinuously re-applied to the mirror surface to replace that washed off by the handpiece spray. The DA can help to keep the surface wet by using the air—water syringe. This is best achieved by her dripping water onto the mirror at the rate of I drop every 3 or 4 seconds (Figure 10.15). Care must be taken that the DA does not release a continuous stream of water, since this will obscure the surface even more. Nor should she hold the syringe tip over the mirror so that it produces a reflection, since this will in itself obscure vision (Figure 10.16). Adequate wetting can be achieved by the DA holding the tip I cm away from the top edge of the mirror. Water slowly dripped from this distance will flow from the top edge across the mirror surface. Where neither of these techniques produces a clear reflection, it is usually because the volume of coolant spray is too high. It should

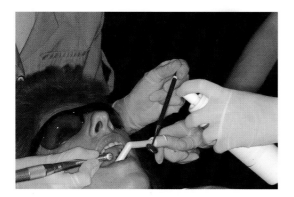

Figure 10.14

The DA spraying the mirror surface with a wetting agent.

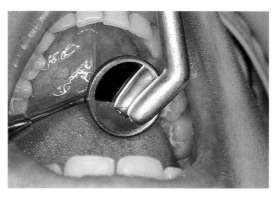

Figure 10.16

The DA obscuring the dentist's view in the mirror by holding the syringe tip too far over its surface.

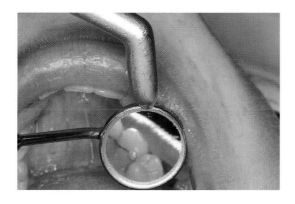

Figure 10.15

The DA dripping water onto the pre-wetted mirror to provide a perfect reflecting surface.

therefore be adjusted to a lower level concomitant with adequate cooling of the bur.

Mirror specifications

- The mirror head should be of a small diameter. This provides less surface area on which spray may fall yet gives an adequate area of mirror to view the tooth. It also has the advantage of leaving more room in the mouth for both dentist and DA to place their other instruments and helps to obtain better vision of the working point.
- The angle of the front surface of the mirror to the long axis of the handle should be 135°. Such an angle will provide a reflecting surface parallel to the tooth surface while allowing the forearm and hand to be held in the correct position (Figure 10.17). Angles significantly greater than 135° will cause the dentist to over-abduct his arm in an attempt to maintain the mirror surface horizontal.
- The handle should be light in weight since a heavy handle places unnecessary strain on the hand and forearm. A mirror is not an operating instrument and can be held with a light grip.

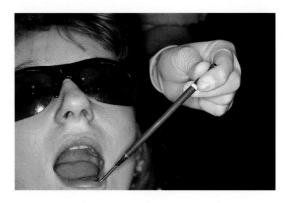

Figure 10.17

Correct grasp for a mirror. The handle is held at its extreme end between the thumb and index finger.

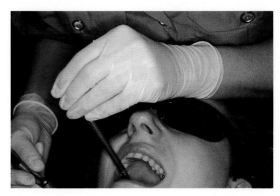

Figure 10.19

The dentist has placed all four fingers on the mirror handle to achieve extra retraction force.

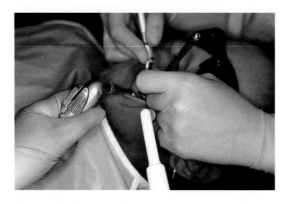

Figure 10.18

Incorrect grasp for a mirror. It is held too far down the handle and obscures the DA's view of the mouth.

The dentist should hold the mirror handle at its extreme end by placing it between the thumb and index finger and resting the handle on the dorsal surface of the middle finger (Figure 10.17). The common practice of holding the mirror handle at its mirror end occurs because most dentists use the left hand to retract soft tissue as well as to hold the mirror. This totally blocks the DA's vision (Figure 10.18) and causes her to work in a distorted posture if she is to see into the mouth. It must be pointed out that the practice is quite unnecessary because a mirror is not an operating instrument and so does not need a finger rest. Holding the mirror at the top of the handle removes the dentist's hand from the DA's sight line and ensures that she can work in a correct posture (Figure 10.17).

For the patient with particularly strong oral musculature it may be more advantageous to use a large diameter mirror, but this is only for use as a tissue retractor and not for viewing. It may also be necessary in such cases to obtain a more rigid grip of the mirror by holding it with all four fingers (Figure 10.19). In this situation, the mirror is in fact being used as an operating instrument.

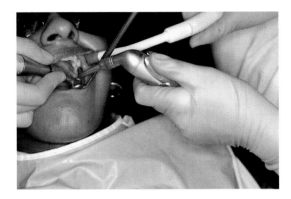

Figure 10.20

Maintaining vision of the cavity. The DA blowing water, then air, onto the cavity.

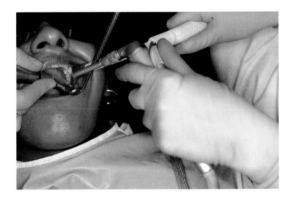

Figure 10.21

The DA slightly rotates her wrist to blow water, then air, onto the mirror surface.

Removal of debris and saliva

Debris and saliva must be continuously removed from the preparation, both intra- or extra-coronal, in order to give the dentist a perfect view of the operating point at all times.

Method

The DA uses the air–water syringe to wash the cavity or preparation and clear it of debris. She then blows air onto it to dry it and so give the dentist a clear view of the progress of the preparation. An accurate assessment is not possible if the operating point is wet. However, when mirror vision is being used, the debris and water invariably will be blown onto the surface of the mirror. As this will obscure the dentist's view, the DA must then wash the mirror to maintain the surface free of debris. The sequence is therefore as follows:

- Wash the cavity with spray.
- Dry the cavity.
- Wash the mirror with a water jet.
- Re-apply wetting agent frequently.

This mirror technique can therefore be seen to be a systematic alternation of water, then air, onto the cavity site, followed by water onto the mirror. Only a slight rotation of the DA's wrist is required to redirect the point of the syringe from the cavity onto the mirror (Figures 10.20–10.21).

If the mirror is not washed continuously as the preparation progresses, debris will dry onto the surface and is then extremely difficult to remove. Should this occur, the mirror must be immediately exchanged for a clean, pre-wetted one to save the break in concentration which will occur if time is spent trying to wash and clean it of debris.

11 Instrument handling

Correct instrument handling is one of the more important factors in reducing stress while increasing efficiency. It allows the dentist to:

- Maintain correct working postures
- Keep his concentration on the working point
- Reduce constant re-accommodation
- Work more efficiently
- Minimize stress

The principle on which this is based is that all instruments and materials should be brought directly to the dentist throughout operative procedures without his attention being diverted from the operating point. This minimizes not only constant operator eye movement away from the working point but also breaks in concentration—both of which are causative factors of mental fatigue.

Rules

For the DA

All instruments must be:

- Located in the DA's working area within her arm's reach
- Held in the DA's left hand
- Held at the non-working end
- Presented with the working end of the instrument pointing in the direction of use
- Passed within the 'transfer zone' (see below)
- Passed in correct sequence of use
- Delivered to the dentist so that the instrument is ready for him to hold by simply opening and closing his grip
- Able to be used by the dentist immediately without him needing to regrasp

For the dentist

- He should hold his hand and fingers in the open position ready to receive the instrument in the correct grasp (see Figure 11.7)
- He must discipline himself always to return the instrument to the DA and *not* discard it on his own working surface

The transfer zone

The 'transfer zone' is an area where the DA's left hand and the dentist's right hand intersect when the forearm is moved naturally, pivoting at the elbow, to the patient's midsagittal plane. It is located over the suprasternal notch and chin of a supine patient (Figure 11.1).

This zone is the ideal one in which to transfer instruments and materials and is the area nearest to the patient's mouth which is not within his line of vision over any part of his face; the risk of trauma is thus reduced.

Instrument handling

There are four phases:

- Grasp—by the dentist
- Pre-delivery—the DA's grasp and presentation
- Delivery—by the DA, used when only a single instrument is involved
- Exchange between the dentist and the DA when two instruments are involved—delivery and exchange are discussed fully in this chapter

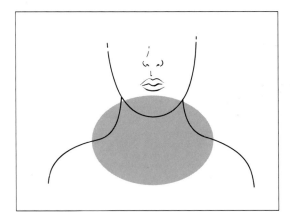

Figure 11.1

The area demarcating the 'transfer zone'.

Dentist's grasp

The four main ones are:

● Pen grasp
● Palm grasp
● Palm–thumb grasp
● Reverse palm–thumb grasp

Pen grasp

This is the one most commonly used and is a similar grasp to that used when holding a pen (Figure 11.2). The instrument is held between the thumb and index finger with the middle finger below to act as a support. Most dentists grasp hand instruments about two-thirds along the shaft towards the working end.

Palm grasp

The instrument is held in the palm of the hand with the last three fingers curved completely around the shaft, the index finger curled some two-thirds around and the thumb extended along the shaft in the direction of the working end. This grasp is most commonly used for forceps and the air–water syringe (Figure 11.3).

Palm–thumb grasp

The instrument is grasped in the palm but with all four fingers curled right around the shaft and the thumb extended along the shaft much nearer to the working end to act as a finger-rest and a guiding plane. This grasp is most commonly used for chisels and excavators (Figure 11.4).

Reverse palm–thumb grasp

This is the most commonly used for rubber-dam clamp forceps and is the grasp used by some operators for extraction forceps. The grasp is similar to the palm–thumb except that the instrument is held in the palm with the working end emerging from below the ulnar border of the hand. The thumb is thus directed along the shaft towards the non-working end.

Pre-delivery

The best delivery grasp for the DA to use in presenting hand instruments to the dentist is the two-fingered one, in which the instrument is held between her thumb and index finger, with the middle finger flexed to place the dorsal–lateral surface of the distal phalanx beneath the instrument shaft (Figure 11.5). Some DAs use a three-fingered delivery grasp, whereby the instrument is held between the tips of the thumb, and index and middle fingers—the three digits forming an equilateral triangle (Figure 11.6). However, this necessitates the DA hyper-rotating her wrist to maintain the instrument in a correct parallel relationship. It is not the method of choice since it distorts the

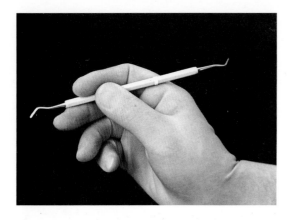

Figure 11.2

A hand instrument held in a pen grasp.

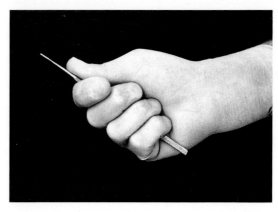

Figure 11.4

A chisel held in a palm–thumb grasp.

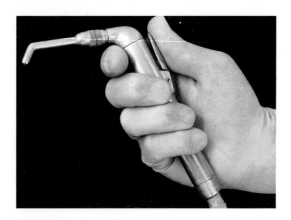

Figure 11.3

An air–water syringe held in a palm grasp.

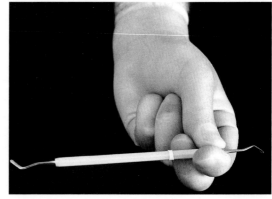

Figure 11.5

The DA presenting a hand instrument, holding it in the two-fingered grasp. Her fingers and wrist are relaxed.

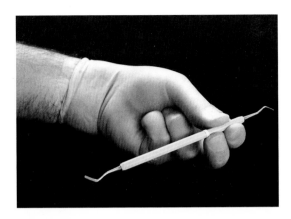

Figure 11.6

The DA presenting a hand instrument using a three-fingered grasp. Although the wrist is not distorted, the instrument is not being presented in the correct parallel relationship to the mouth. To do so would necessitate a severe bending of the wrist.

wrist, places too much pressure on the thumb to maintain the position and is tiring to the hand.

The two-fingered delivery grasp is preferred because it gives support along the long length of the instrument shaft and allows the wrist to assume a more natural position while still presenting the instrument parallel to the dentist's frontal plane.

The DA holds the instrument (Figure 11.7):

- In her left hand
- At its non-working end
- With the working end pointing in the direction of use
- In the transfer zone
- With the instrument shaft parallel to the dentist's frontal plane

Delivery

One of the fundamentals of good assisting is that every instrument must be delivered to the dentist in such a way that, simply by tightening his fingers on it, he will be holding it correctly, and can use it immediately without needing to change his finger position. It is therefore essential that the dentist holds his hand in the precise pre-grasp position with his fingers open and ready to receive the instrument from the DA.

Perhaps the most fundamental principle of instrument transfer is that the DA must deliver the hand instrument *to* the dentist, rather than the dentist taking the instrument *from* the DA.

Instrument transfer techniques

Direct placement

When the dentist starts without any instrument in his hand, an instrument can be placed directly into his hand by the DA. This is the simplest and most basic delivery sequence.

Some examples of direct placement follow. The pre-delivery and delivery sequence of hypodermic syringes is fully described on pages 162–4.

Plastic filling instruments

These are mostly held in a pen grasp, but a palm–thumb grasp is also used occasionally.

Pen grasp

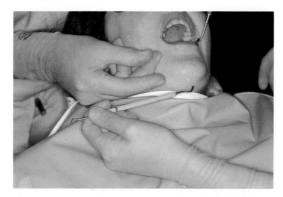

Figure 11.7

Pre-delivery: The DA holds the instrument in the two-fingered delivery position. The dentist holds his hand to the right of the patient's face with his fingers open in the receiving position for a pen grasp. He maintains his hand in this position while the DA places the instrument in it.

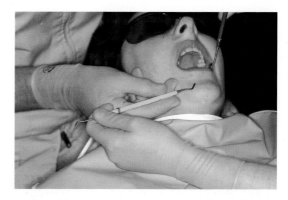

Figure 11.8

Delivery: The DA moves the instrument towards the dentist's open fingers and thumb and, with a slightly downward and forward movement of her left hand, places the instrument firmly into the dentist's open fingers.

Palm–thumb grasp

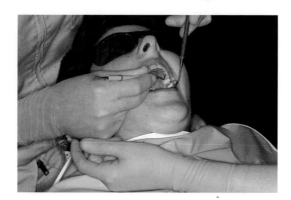

Figure 11.9

The dentist tightens his fingers and the DA releases her grasp on the instrument. It is now ready for immediate use in the correct working grasp.

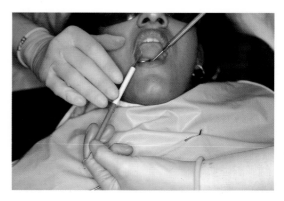

Figure 11.10

The procedures are the same as for the pen grasp except that the dentist must hold his hand open in the correct receiving position for a palm–thumb grasp. The DA places the instrument directly into the dentist's open palm.

Mirror and probe

The need for the dentist to hold the mirror at the end of the handle has already been stressed (see page 114). The probe, however, is held in a normal pen grasp near its working end. The delivery must therefore be such as to ensure that the dentist receives each of these instruments in a slightly different grasp.

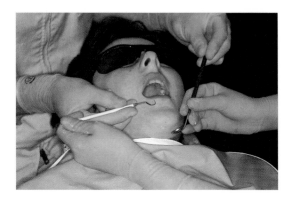

Figure 11.11

Pre-delivery: The DA holds the probe in her left hand near its non-working end and the mirror in her right hand with the thumb and first two fingers mid-way along the handle. The presence of her fingers in this position on the mirror ensures that the dentist cannot hold the mirror in the middle of its handle and must grasp the only part available to him—the extreme end.

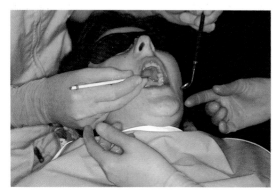

Figure 11.12

Delivery: With the shafts of these instruments at approximately 45° to the dorsum of her hands, and the non-working ends pointing towards the dentist's chest, the DA places them directly into his open finger-rest and releases her grasp. The dentist now has the mirror and probe in correct, though different, grasps.

Tweezers

A pen grasp is used.

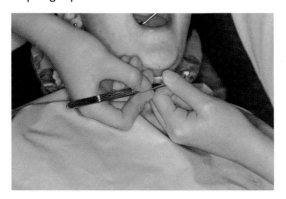

Figure 11.13

Pre-delivery: If non-locking tweezers are being used to hold an object, for example a cotton pledget, the DA must grip them near to the working end to keep the beaks (points) firmly together to hold the object. The dentist is then able to grasp them when she releases her grip. If locking tweezers are used, the DA grips these at their non-working end because the beaks are already pre-locked onto the object. **Delivery**: With both non-locking and locking tweezers, this is the same as that described for delivery of a plastic filling instrument.

Amalgam carrier

There are two grasps which can be used: the palm–finger grasp and the thumb–finger grasp. The choice of which of these grasps to use depends purely on the personal preference of the dentist.

Palm–finger grasp

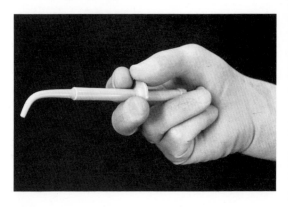

Figure 11.14

The barrel of the carrier is held between the dentist's index and middle fingers, with the plunger end on the *ball* of his thumb (thenar eminence).

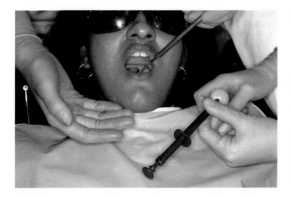

Figure 11.15

Pre-delivery: The receptacle containing the mixed amalgam is held in the DA's right hand. The amalgam carrier is held near the nozzle end between the thumb and index finger of her left hand and is supported by the middle phalanx of the middle finger beneath the shaft and by the thumb along the top of the shaft. The loaded carrier is moved towards the dentist with the nozzle pointing upwards for a maxillary cavity and downwards for a mandibular cavity.

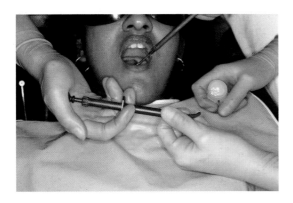

Figure 11.16

Delivery: The DA applies pressure from her thumb on the medial side of the carrier, drops her index finger and moves the carrier through 45° with a rolling movement of the thumb over the index finger. The long axis now points towards the dentist's right hand and the DA presses the plunger firmly onto the ball of his thumb, with the barrel crossing his palm from the tip of the middle finger to the base of the thumb.

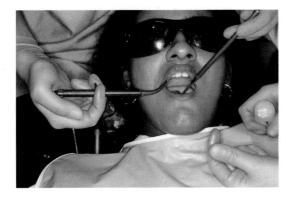

Figure 11.17

The dentist only has to close his palm and fingers to obtain a firm grasp and carry the amalgam carrier into the patient's mouth.

Thumb–finger grasp

The barrel is held between the index and middle fingers, with the plunger end placed on the pad of the thumb (distal phalanx). This is similar to the grasp used to hold an aspirating hypodermic syringe (see page 164).

Pre-delivery and delivery: The carrier is loaded and presented as described for the palm grasp but the shaft is moved through only 30° to place the plunger end on the pad of the dentist's thumb and the shaft between his fingers. The smaller movement is needed because the pad is nearer than the ball of the thumb.

Amalgam placement by the DA

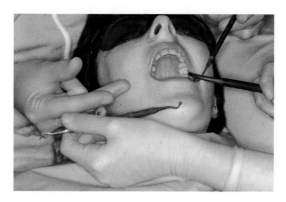

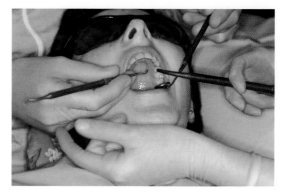

Figure 11.18

Wherever possible, the DA should place amalgam directly into the cavity instead of passing a loaded carrier to the dentist. This saves a great deal of carrier–instrument exchange and allows the dentist to retain the packing instrument in his right hand. When this technique is used, the DA loads the carrier, picks up the first packer in the sequence and places it directly into the dentist's right hand.

Figure 11.19

Holding the carrier in her right hand, she then feeds the amalgam directly into the cavity.

Most DAs find it easier to load the amalgam carrier from an amalgam receptacle placed on their work surface. The disadvantage is that the DA has to move away from the patient's mouth to her work surface every time she reloads the carrier. Other DAs prefer to hold both the receptacle and the packer in their left hand, which eliminates the problem but conversely makes it more difficult to exchange packers. Moreover, in exchanging packers, the DA may inadvertently rotate her hand and spill the amalgam.

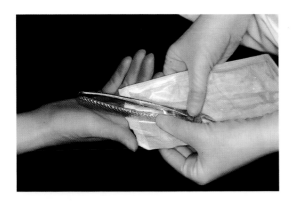

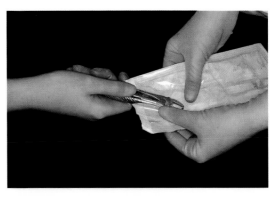

Figure 11.20

Delivery: Gripping the end of the bag between her left thumb and fingers with palm facing upwards, the DA presents the handles of the forceps to the dentist, whose hand is extended in an open palm grasp.

Figure 11.21

The DA places the handles directly into the middle of his palm, and he then closes his palm over the handles and draws the forceps out of the bag. This technique ensures that the DA's hands are in contact only with the outside of the sterile bag throughout the entire sequence.

Extraction forceps

All forceps and surgical instruments must be kept sealed in their sterile bag until immediately prior to use. Their working ends must never be handled by the DA and the following placement technique must therefore be followed to ensure this.

Pre-delivery: The DA opens the sterile bag at its handle end and, holding the bag over the beaks of the forceps with one hand, manipulates the instrument with the other so that approximately one-third of the shaft protrudes from the open end.

Exchange of instruments

When the dentist requires the next instrument in a working sequence, it must be exchanged for the one that has been in use. To this the term 'instrument exchange' is applied.

Principles

- The DA must anticipate the dentist's requirements by knowing which instrument he needs next in any given operating procedure.
- A rationalized and logical work sequence of instrumentation for each procedure must be established between the dentist and the DA and thereafter followed by the dentist.
- The dentist must indicate that he has finished using the first instrument by lifting its working end away from the tooth and moving it just out of the mouth, all the time maintaining the instrument at the same angle as the one at which it has been held while in use (Figure 11.22).
- This action acts as a signal to the DA that the next instrument is required and she should make the initial movement necessary for a smooth exchange. It must be emphasized that the dentist must not move the used instrument more than 2 cm out of the mouth and it should be held in that position until the DA takes it.

Methods of instrument exchange

There are four methods of instrument exchange. In each of the following descriptions, the used instrument will be referred to as 'A' and is coded yellow; the new instrument is 'B', coded red.

- Take and place
- Parallel exchange
- Combined take and place with parallel exchange
- Change of operator grasp

Take and place

This exchange can only be used if the DA has both hands free (Figures 11.23–11.27).

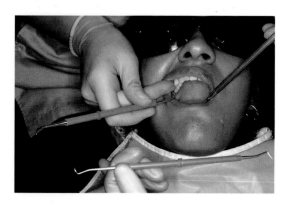

Figure 11.22

The dentist signals he has finished with an instrument by moving it 2 cm out of the mouth. The DA holds the next instrument ready in the transfer zone.

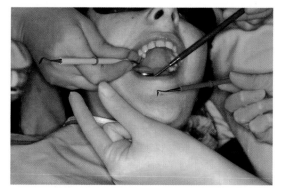

Figure 11.23

Pre-delivery: Instrument B is held in the DA's right hand at its working end and to the right side of the patient's chin. The DA's hand is placed in the receiving position just to the left of the dentist's right hand and with the thumb and index finger open ready to receive instrument A.

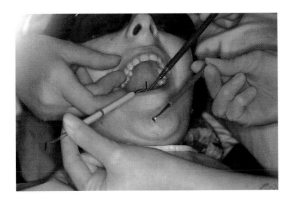

Figure 11.24

Exchange: The DA grasps A at its non-working end and the dentist releases his grasp, allowing the instrument to be removed by the DA.

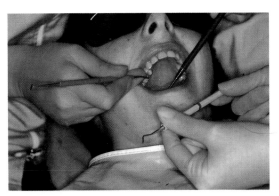

Figure 11.26

The dentist moves B into the mouth while the DA moves A across from her left hand into her right thumb and index finger.

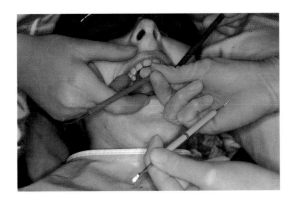

Figure 11.25

At the same time as the DA removes A, she moves B across from right to left into the transfer zone, placing it directly into the dentist's open fingers, and releases her grip.

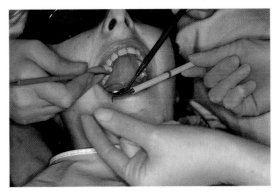

Figure 11.27

The DA retains her left hand in position to receive back instrument B when the dentist has finished.

Should the dentist require to use instrument A once more, the DA has it ready for exchange in exactly the same sequence. The movement of the two instruments describes an elliptical path with a smooth, easy action and no crossing over of either the dentist's or the DA's hands.

Parallel exchange

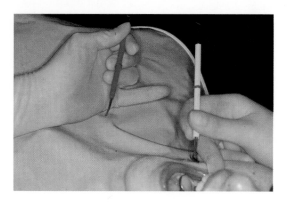

Figure 11.28

Pre-delivery: The DA holds B in her left hand at its non-working end, with the shaft parallel to A, and extends her little finger. At this stage it should be approximately 6 cm away from A, with the working end pointing in the direction of use. The dentist signals for exchange to begin by moving A 2 cm out of the mouth.

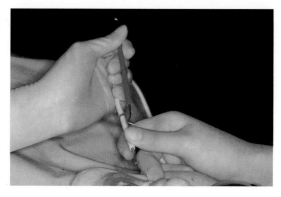

Figure 11.30

Exchange: The DA grips instrument A firmly around its shaft at its non-working end with her little finger.

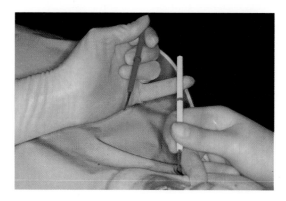

Figure 11.29

The DA extends the little finger of her left hand, placing it beneath the non-working end of A.

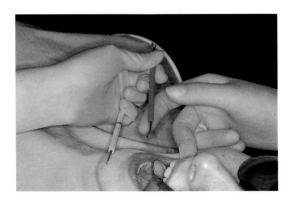

Figure 11.31

The dentist releases his grasp, but maintains his hand in the same position, and the DA removes instrument A. At the same time she moves B towards the mouth, over A, keeping B parallel at all times. This is achieved by a slight downward drop of the DA's hand, advancing her left thumb and index finger towards the dentist's hand.

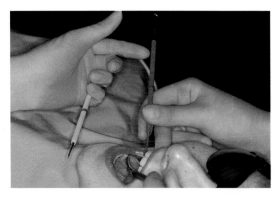

Figure 11.33

The DA releases her grip and the dentist tightens his grasp on instrument B, ready for immediate use and moves it into the patient's mouth.

This exchange method is the one used most frequently. It is simple, rapid, easily learned and does not produce distortion of the DA's hand or wrist, or tangling of instruments. It can be used for all instruments and handpieces, but is principally employed to exchange hand instruments.

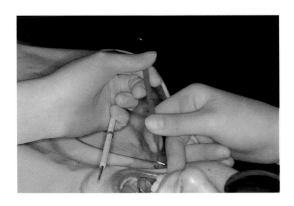

Figure 11.32

The movement is maintained until the instrument is firmly placed into the dentist's open fingers.

Combined take and place with parallel exchange

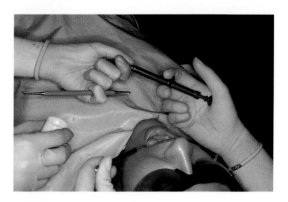

Figure 11.34

Pre-delivery: The DA places the first amalgam packer with its non-working end in the little finger of her left hand, puts the amalgam receptacle in her right and loads the carrier by holding it in her left hand approximately one-third along its shaft from the nozzle end.

Exchange: The carrier is directly placed into the dentist's hand in palm-finger grasp as previously described but with the packer still being held in the DA's little finger.

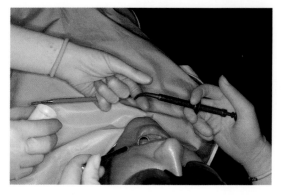

Figure 11.36

The dentist moves the carrier out of the mouth and the DA takes it from him by holding it at its nozzle end.

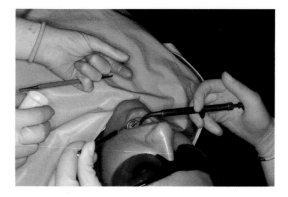

Figure 11.35

The dentist places the amalgam, while the DA maintains her left hand in the transfer zone.

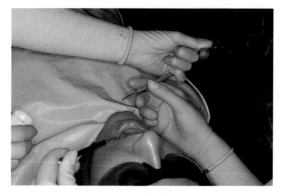

Figure 11.37

Having firmly grasped the carrier, the DA raises her left hand by approximately 8 cm, placing the packer at the level of the dentist's open pen grasp. The DA places the packer directly into the dentist's right hand.

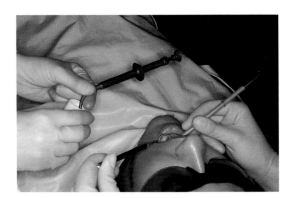

Figure 11.38

The DA reloads the carrier while the dentist uses the packer to condense the amalgam.

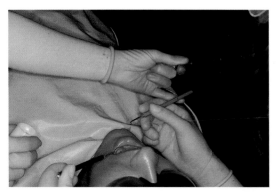

Figure 11.39

The refilled carrier is presented. The DA removes the packer by grasping it in her little finger and places the carrier into the dentist's hand, as shown in Figure 11.34.

While the dentist feeds the next amalgam increment into the cavity, the DA retains the packer in her fifth finger in the transfer zone ready to re-present it. It should be noted that no change of the DA's grip is necessary with this technique.

Change of operator grasp

Occasionally the dentist may have to exchange an instrument he is using in a pen grasp for a second instrument which has to be held in a palm–thumb grasp.

Exchange: The DA uses her left hand to remove the instrument being used in the pen grasp (instrument A), as though she were beginning the sequence for parallel exchange.

Having moved instrument A, the DA does not at this point place instrument B into the dentist's open fingers but instead holds it in the transfer zone. During this pause, the dentist rotates his hand through 90° to place it in the open palm–thumb grasp position. The DA then rotates B through 45° so that its working end points upwards in the direction of the patient's mouth.

The DA moves the shaft of B into a vertical position and places it directly into the dentist's palm–thumb grasp (see Figure 11.10).

Though not a common situation, this change of grasp technique illustrates the importance of correct hand movements and finger positions by the dentist in giving clear guidance to the DA; they are thus a prerequisite of good instrument exchange.

Faults in instrument exchange

- The DA holds instrument B (yellow) at the working end (Figure 11.40). This places the non-working end into the dentist's hand (Figure 11.41) and he is forced to regrasp the instrument by moving his thumb and forefinger along the shaft to the working end, in order to achieve the correct pen grasp.
- Instrument B is not presented parallel to the dentist's frontal plane, that is, pointing towards him. This necessitates the dentist twisting his wrist in order to grasp the instrument correctly (Figure 11.42).
- Instead of moving instrument A (blue) out of the mouth and keeping it parallel, the dentist rotates the instrument and points it towards the DA (Figure 11.43). This places A in the wrong relationship to B (yellow) for a satisfactory parallel exchange to be achieved. In order to exchange instruments the DA is required to distort her wrist severely (Figure 11.44).

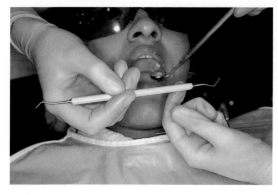

Figure 11.41

The dentist is forced to grasp the instrument at its non-working end, necessitating a change of grasp before he can use it.

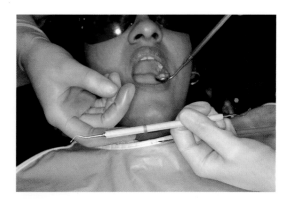

Figure 11.40

Faults in instrument exchange (1)
The DA presents instrument B, but holds it at its working end.

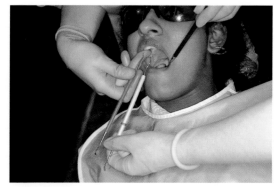

Figure 11.42

Faults in instrument exchange (2)
The DA presents instrument B pointing towards the dentist instead of parallel to his frontal plane. Parallel exhange can only be achieved if the dentist severely distorts his wrist.

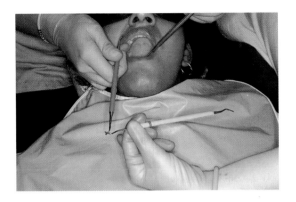

Figure 11.43

Faults in instrument exchange (3)
The dentist rotates instrument A towards the DA.

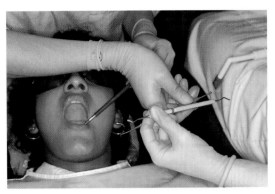

Figure 11.45

Faults in instrument exchange (4)
The DA holds the instrument too near to her body, causing the dentist to over-extend his right arm.

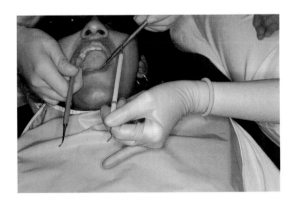

Figure 11.44

Parallel exchange of the two instruments can only be achieved if the DA severely distorts her wrist.

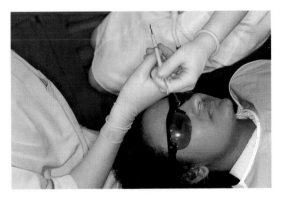

Figure 11.46

Faults in instrument exchange (5)
The dentist moves the instrument towards him, causing transfer to take place over the patient's eyes.

This fault is perhaps the most common one and the cause is often two-fold. Firstly, the dentist mistakenly believes that it is easier for the DA to grasp the instrument if he rotates it and points it at her. Secondly, the DA compounds the error by not holding B near enough to the patient's mouth and parallel to A.

- The DA does not hold the instrument in the transfer zone. She holds it too near to her body, so that to exchange instruments the dentist is required to over-extend his upper arm and move his right hand across the patient's chest (Figure 11.45).
- The dentist moves instrument A out of the mouth and to the right, placing it too near his own body. To exchange instruments, the DA has to reach across the patient's chest, moving her hand into the dentist's working area and producing over-extension of her upper arm.
- Prior to exchange, the dentist moves instrument A upwards and towards him, instead of away from him. This causes instrument exchange to take place over the patient's face (Figure 11.46). This is hazardous because of the danger that an instrument may be dropped onto the patient's face or that the sharp end of an instrument may cause trauma.

12   Cross-infection control

This chapter offers basic practical guidelines on cross-infection control. Hypodermic needles, matrix bands, burs and many hand instruments (particularly scalers) often break the oral epithelium, and blood, which may contain pathogenic micro-organisms, can contaminate the dentist's hands, instruments and working surfaces. It is essential that everything which has been contaminated with blood or saliva is sterilized to prevent the risk of transmission of infection to the next patient, the dentist or the DA (Wood and Martin, 1989). In addition the increasing incidence of AIDS and hepatitis B makes it inevitable that a number of dentists are already treating patients who are carriers of HIV or hepatitis B virus (HBV) but who are unaware of it or unwilling to disclose it. It is likely that the number of such patients will increase in future years.

For these reasons, it is more important than ever for the dental profession to improve cross-infection control in the practice. In a perfect world, a totally aseptic environment would be ideal but this can never really be achieved in a general dental practice. However, the highest possible levels of cross-infection control must be achieved by using all the modern methods available to dentists. These will reduce the level of pathogens in the practice, particularly in the treatment area, so protecting not only the dentist and his staff but also patients— particularly those whose immune systems are compromised.

Definitions

- *Sterilization* is defined as 'the complete destruction of all living matter' (Wilson, 1984).

- *Disinfection* refers to the destruction of pathogens only (Wilson, 1984), indicating the destruction or removal of all organisms capable of giving rise to infection.
- *Antisepsis* refers to the prevention of infection, usually by inhibiting growth of bacteria.

Criteria for sterilization procedures

Sterilization procedures for use in general dental practice must:

- Destroy all micro-organisms and their spores
- Be meticulously observed
- Be easy to apply and effect
- Not cause damage to instruments

Staff must be given sufficient time to allow them to carry out procedures properly, and an adequate supply of instruments and containers must be readily available. This entails duplication, particularly of those instruments used most frequently.

Infecting organisms

Those of most concern to the dental practitioner are bacteria, viruses and fungi.

Bacteria

Most pathogenic bacteria can reproduce very rapidly by cell division and can produce active infection. Some are able to produce spores which,

135

though metabolically inactive, can survive long periods before the appropriate environment triggers germination to a new and infective phase. The spores are much more difficult to destroy than the actual bacteria and the ideal sterilization procedure must therefore be capable of destroying not only bacteria but spores as well.

Viruses

These are small infectious agents, only visible with an electron microscope. They possess a genome of nucleic acid, which reproduces inside living cells and is not affected by antibiotics. Fortunately viruses are much less robust than bacteria and can be destroyed by high temperatures and disinfectants. However, some are very resistant, such as herpes which is resistant to both disinfection and low temperature. It has been known to remain infectious after drying on work surfaces for several days and to survive temperatures of 60 °C/140 °F for 4 hours. A multiple cross-infection strategy is therefore needed to restrict or eliminate virus transmission.

Fungi

Many fungi can cause oral diseases, and in dentistry the most common one is the yeast *Candida albicans*. Under appropriate conditions, it can become pathogenic (giving rise for example to oral thrush). It must be noted that fungi also produce spores which are highly resistant to most methods of sterilization.

Cross-infection in dentistry

Infectious agents can be spread by:

● A parenteral route (for example, HBV).
● Direct contact (for example herpes simplex virus).
● Inert objects such as dental hand instruments. Other inert transmitters include work surfaces,

handles on drawers and lights, and chair controls. Cross-infection can be produced by the contamination of one inert surface by another, for example a non-sterile instrument placed on a work surface or in a drawer renders that surface or drawer non-sterile and contaminated with micro-organisms. These may then be transmitted to the next patient.
● Aerosols—small droplets suspended in air—principally produced by turbines, ultrasonic scalers and three-in-one syringes. Aerosols thus created can remain present in the air for a considerable time and so contamination can be passed on from one patient to another.
● Splatter—larger droplets which are usually visible to the naked eye.

Guidelines for control

Total *surgical* sterility is rarely practicable in the general dental practice. A sensible and practical regime should be followed by taking those basic precautions by which all methods of transmission can be eliminated.

Patient cooperation

Display a notice asking patients to inform the dentist of any changes in medical status or drug therapy.

Medical history

Take a careful medical history (Figure 12.1), with particular attention to any history of jaundice, blood transfusions or of regular visits abroad in the

Figure 12.1

An example of a medical history form.

PATIENT'S NAME ....

| PLEASE READ THIS QUESTIONNAIRE AND TICK THE ANSWER TO EACH QUESTION | YES | NO |

PLEASE READ THIS QUESTIONNAIRE AND TICK THE ANSWER TO EACH QUESTION YES NO

1) Have you had any serious illness or operation especially during the last 12 months? [ ] [ ]

2) Do you have or have you had any of the following?
    a) Heart conditions of any kind [ ] [ ]
    b) High blood pressure [ ] [ ]
    c) Rheumatic fever or rheumatic heart disease [ ] [ ]
    d) Congenital heart disease [ ] [ ]
    e) Asthma [ ] [ ]
    f) Fainting spells or blackouts [ ] [ ]
    g) Diabetes [ ] [ ]
    h) Tuberculosis [ ] [ ]
    i) Hepatitis [ ] [ ]

3) Have you had any other serious illness? [ ] [ ]

4) Do you have any blood disorders such as anaemia? [ ] [ ]

5) Have you had any abnormal bleeding associated with previous operations or dental extractions? [ ] [ ]

6) Are you taking or have you taken any of the following during the last 12 months?
    a) Antibiotics [ ] [ ]
    b) Anticoagulants [ ] [ ]
    c) Tablets for high blood pressure [ ] [ ]
    d) Cortisone (steroids) [ ] [ ]
    e) Tablets for nerves or depression [ ] [ ]
    f) Tranquillizers [ ] [ ]
    g) Insulin [ ] [ ]
    h) Digitalis [ ] [ ]

7) Have you had any allergic or abnormal reactions to any of the following?
    a) Local anaesthesia [ ] [ ]
    b) Aspirin [ ] [ ]
    c) Penicillin or any antibiotics [ ] [ ]
    d) Any other drug or food [ ] [ ]

8) Have you had any complication during dental treatment in the past? [ ] [ ]

9) If you are pregnant, please tell us the expected date of birth. ....

10) Are you a registered addictive drug user? [ ] [ ]

11) CHILD ATTENDING FOR THE FIRST TIME:
Does the child bruise easily and/or has the child taken aspirin recently as a pain killer? [ ] [ ]

12) Have you had HEPATITIS at any time or have you been informed that
you are a hepatitis carrier? [ ] [ ]

13) If you believe that you may have had contact with someone who is HIV positive, or a confirmed
AIDS carrier, or if there is any doubt about your own status, please indicate that you would like
a talk in the strictest confidence with one of our dentists.
You will not be discriminated against in any way if there is a positive condition known but it is
essential that we are informed. [ ] [ ]

SIGNATURE .... DATE ....

recent past. This must be updated at every recall examination to ensure there has been no change in medical history.

The medical history questionnaire shown in Figure 12.1 has questions specifically asking about hepatitis and HIV. This is a most important responsibility, which dentists must not ignore.

The other important point to be emphasized is that the form must be signed by the patient so that there is no possibility of legal problems at a later date.

Suction

Use high-speed suction intra-orally. This will considerably reduce both splatter and aerosol transmission.

Protective spectacles

The dentist, DA and patient must all wear protective spectacles (see page 94). These will prevent mechanical irritation of the eyes, in particular from debris produced by cavity preparations, scaling or prophylaxis, and will prevent ocular infection from organisms such as herpes—an unpleasant condition that is difficult to treat.

Masks

Masks should be worn by both dentist and DA. These afford very effective protection from inhalation of aerosols.

The best type of mask is a solid one made of fibre. However, if the fibre is too densely packed, the passage of air is impeded and the wearer may find it uncomfortable when worn for long periods. One manufacturer has overcome this problem by applying an electrostatic charge to the fibre, which gives a higher bacteria-trapping efficiency with less-densely packed fibre and so allows easier breathing. This type is said to filter 99 per cent of bacteria of the particle size normally found in exhaled breath and 95 per cent of those in aerosols.

Tray system

A sterile tray system must be used (see pages 151–3) which confines all contaminated instruments and

materials to a single tray. Failing this, all trays and working surfaces should be covered with an impervious disposable cover. After each patient, this cover can be used to wrap the contaminated instruments prior to their removal.

Disinfection of surfaces

All surfaces should be disinfected with one of the many hard-surface disinfectants available. These could be 1 per cent hypochlorite, gluteraldehyde or iodophores.

During the course of the day, all buttons, handles and switches must be cleaned between patients, using one of the many disinfecting sprays available. Ideally disinfectant should be sprayed onto surfaces, wiped off and then re-applied without any further wiping. This dilutes the number of micro-organisms present and also ensures a high level of disinfection.

Handles must be covered with foil or transparent plastic wrap and light-curing tips should be covered with transparent cling-film (see page 146).

The need for frequent cleaning and disinfecting of the surfaces can be reduced by applying a zoning system. This involves the use of coloured tape to demarcate a minimal number of areas of the work surfaces as work zones. All instruments and materials should be restricted to these zones. This procedure reduces the number of areas contaminated each time a patient is treated and so restricts the movement of infected material during clinical procedures.

At the end of the day all surfaces should be cleaned with a 1 per cent (w/v) hypochlorite or 2 per cent (w/v) gluteraldehyde solution. All floors and dental units should be similarly treated.

Gloves

Hands are the primary vehicle for the transmission of cross-infection and gloves are a simple and effective barrier against this.

In a study of a group of 15 dentists who had contracted HBV, it was found that none had worn gloves (Martin, 1988). All bitterly regretted this, as in every case the hands were the most likely route for ingress of the virus. The study also found that chlorhexidine has no action on HBV so that washing with it offers no protection against the virus. The use of gloves is therefore mandatory for both dentist and DA.

Gloves should be thin enough to provide adequate tactile sense for the dentist yet strong enough not to tear easily. They should fit the hand very well. Authorities differ in their attitude to whether gloves should be washed or not. In the USA, the Centers for Disease Control does not accept the repeated use of the same pair of gloves by disinfecting them between patients (ADA Council on Dental Materials, Dental Practice and Therapeutics, 1988). However, most authorities in the UK will accept this procedure, provided the gloves are of the type of material which will stand up to frequent washing without becoming sticky. There are gloves available which meet this criterion and may also have a bactericidal effect themselves.

The wear characteristics of latex gloves are not so different from those of natural skin. They will harden, soften, abrade, flake and split if not treated correctly, so reducing their efficiency as a guard against cross-infection. Bar and liquid soap and hot water should never be used for either hand or glove disinfection. Such washing materials do not disinfect adequately, are unkind to the skin and cause the latex to deteriorate when applied frequently. Anatriptic alcohol hand-rubs combined with the use of cold water and non-soap wash lotions provide the best system. Any alcohol hand-rub solution should contain additives to restore the natural oil of the skin.

Ideally, a fresh pair of gloves should be used for each patient. However, this is now recognized as being very expensive and the tendency is to re-use them. If gloves are not changed after every patient, they should certainly be changed if a puncture is suspected and before and after surgical or any other cases which have resulted in blood contamination. Autoclavable gloves are now being developed to overcome this problem of re-use.

It has been repeatedly shown that a percentage of all types of glove shows some defect. The rate varies between 1.7 and 9 per cent (*Clinical Research Associates Newsletter*, 1985). It is therefore important for each pair of gloves to be tested by the operator before use. This can be done quickly by inflating the glove and observing whether any defects are apparent.

Prior to donning gloves, any cuts should be covered with a plaster.

Hands and nails should be scrubbed with a surgical hand scrub and dried on a single-use disposable towel. Between every patient, gloved hands should be scrubbed and washed with a similar scrub. These have a broad disinfectant action including anti-HBV and anti-HIV.

Disposable equipment

Disposable items should be used wherever possible since this obviates the need for sterilization and reduces the chance of cross-infection.

Such items currently available include:

- Hypodermic and suturing needles, cartridges and scalpel blades
- Mouthwash cups (stored in a sealed, wall-mounted dispenser)
- Saliva ejector tips
- Bibs—these should have an upper absorbent layer and a plastic lower layer
- X-ray tabs
- Vacuum tips
- Impression trays
- Dappens pots
- Hand towels—these should preferably be disposable but failing this they should be of the roller type which presents a fresh section of towel on each occasion of use

Any sharp disposable items such as surgical and hypodermic needles and scalpel blades must be placed in a 'sharps' box', a rigid container which is sealed before disposal. These containers are supplied and collected by commercial companies or local hospitals.

In dentistry, unlike in medical practice, resheathing of hypodermic needles is usually necessary. When resheathing, it is essential to have adequate protection against needle stab injury and there are many devices on the market which effectively eliminate this possibility (see pages 162–4). For those dentists who prefer not to resheath, there are systems available which remove and dispose of the needle without the necessity to touch it after the injection has been administered.

It is also important to emphasize that suturing needles should not be touched in order to re-grip during use. The risk of glove and skin perforation is considerable.

Impressions

All impressions and bite registrations should be disinfected before sending to the laboratory. Self-sterilizing alginate materials are now available.

X-ray packets

Contaminated X-ray packets must be opened only when wearing gloves.

Aspirators

Aspirators and spitoons should be cleaned and disinfected using one of the new aspirator-cleaning solutions. These are gluteraldehyde-based and are effective against HBV and HIV.

Vaccination

The dentist and *every* member of his staff (including reception staff) must be vaccinated against HBV, tetanus, poliomyelitis and tuberculosis.

Training and review

All staff must be thoroughly trained to understand and effect all practice policies for the prevention of cross-infection. Particular attention must be given to training new members. All procedures must be reviewed periodically to ensure that they are being carried out completely and effectively.

Sterilization procedures

Mechanical cleaning

Whatever method of sterilization is used, it will be ineffective if instruments are not totally free from debris, particularly blood, protein and cement, which would insulate micro-organisms from heat or other sterilization conditions. It is therefore essential that all instruments are mechanically cleaned before any sterilization procedure. Instruments may be washed by hand or may be cleaned by immersion in an ultrasonic bath.

Washing by hand

The instruments first must be soaked in disinfectant, preferably one which contains an agent which will soften or dissolve debris, and then must be physically scrubbed. It is advisable for the DA to wear thick, heavy-duty gloves to protect her from injury and possible infection from sharp edges of instruments.

Ultrasonic cleaning

Ultrasonic cleaning is preferable, being more effective and quicker. This works on the principle that a transducer fixed below a tank filled with fluid transforms electrical energy into mechanical vibratory energy. When the vibrations pass into the fluid, they produce high-frequency sound waves in that fluid. This produces millions of tiny bubbles which implode onto the instrument and displace debris. They penetrate into crevices not normally reached by normal cleaning.

Instruments may be laid directly in the bath, but it is preferable to have them suspended in the fluid since the sound waves are then more efficiently distributed over their entire surface.

The fluid is usually one made specifically for use in the tank. An alternative is to use a good disinfectant which inactivates as many micro-organisms as possible. This reduces the chances of the DA being infected through accidental injury while transferring instruments from the ultrasonic bath to sterilization trays.

The following points should be noted:

- Hand instruments should be placed in a perforated metal container, which is then suspended in the fluid by a frame from the top of the tank.
- Burs, endodontic instruments and other small objects should be placed in a glass beaker containing a fluid specifically made for cleaning them and the beaker similarly suspended.

- Handpieces require a special oily fluid and this should be placed in a suitable container, such as a beaker, and the handpiece immersed directly into it. The oily fluid can be left in the handpiece, provided excess is wiped off prior to use. If handpieces are not ultrasonically cleaned, they must be cleansed on the outside, oiled and then autoclaved.
- Instruments or burs must not be piled on top of each other but laid separately in their container so that the cleaning effect is maximized.
- Fluids must be changed frequently.

It must be emphasized that the ultrasonic bath is purely a mechanical cleaner and does not sterilize the instruments so that, after cleaning, they must be loaded either into autoclaving bags or onto trays, which are then placed in the autoclave or dry-heat oven.

Methods of sterilization

Autoclaving

Autoclaving delivers heat through pressurized steam. Saturated steam condenses on objects cooler than itself and, by giving up its latent heat, quickly raises them to its own temperature.

Over a century ago Koch, Gaffky and Loeffler (1881), carried out the first study of the germicidal action of moist heat. They showed that the temperature required for sterilization is much lower than with dry heat and that steam under pressure is more effective than that at atmospheric pressure. Moist heat also has greater penetrating power. It is now universally recognized that autoclaving is the best method of sterilization in general dental practice, being the only one which can be used for all instruments, handpieces and textiles.

Autoclaving sterilizes by converting water to steam at a temperature of 134°C/273.2°F for 3 minutes under pressures of 2 bar (30 psi). Lower temperatures require longer times (Table 12.1).

There are two basic types of autoclave:

- The small automatic type. This relies on steam entering the chamber by downward displacement of air only.
- The porous-load type, in which air is drawn out of the chamber by a vacuum pump.

The latter is the better of the two systems.

Autoclaving works by hot steam contacting the surface of the instrument and not by heat alone. Any trapped air may prevent steam from contacting parts of the load and thus complete sterilization may not occur. Open sterilization is therefore required. Perforated trays should be used, and glasses or other hollow containers laid on their side. Space must be left between instruments and so the autoclave must not be overloaded. Single instruments such as forceps or other surgical instruments should be sealed in individual clear-view bags with an indicator strip which changes colour when it is sterilized. Time–steam–temperature (TST) strips and Browne tubes (see page 143) must also be used from time to time to check that the sterilizer is working effectively.

Table 12.1 Temperature–time relationships for autoclaving sterilization.

Temperature °C	°F	Time minutes
115–118	239–244.4	30
121–124	249.8–255.2	15
126–129	258.8–264.2	10
134–138	273.2–280.4	3

Economical autoclave

Because of the relatively high cost of even the smallest conventional autoclave suitable for use in general practice, an economical porous-load machine is commercially available which consists of a pressure vessel with a heating element at the bottom and a removable lid.

Air is evacuated through a small pintle in the lid until the whole vessel is filled with steam. When the sterilizing temperature of 126 °C/258.8 °F is achieved, a light comes on and the cycle is automatically held for 11 minutes. If the instruments are immediately required at the end of the cycle, the pressure can be released through the valve on the lid, which can then be removed and the instruments used after 1 minute of cooling. The whole cycle takes around 25 minutes. It is suitable for instruments and handpieces, both of which are held in perforated plastic cassettes inserted vertically into the chamber.

Advantages

- Extremely low cost—there is no excuse for any practitioner not to have an autoclaving system in their practice
- Instruments are dry and available quickly after end of cycle
- Numerous safety features

Disadvantages

- The cycle (25 minutes) is much longer than that of the conventional autoclave (3 minutes)
- Steam is released into the room and this can affect decor
- Tray systems cannot be used

Chemiclave

This type of autoclave is popular in the USA. It incorporates a chamber heating up a mixture of formaldehyde or isopropyl acetone and methylethyl ketone to 130 °C/266 °F for 3 minutes.

Advantages

- Does not cause rusting of instruments
- Use for delicate items such as orthodontic pliers

Disadvantage

- Can emit vapour—a scavenger device should be used

Dry heat

Dry-heat sterilization is usually carried out at 160 °C/320 °F for 1 hour. However, it must be emphasized that the heating up and cooling time can be as much as a further hour. To allow free circulation of air, items should not be placed too closely together on the shelves.

Advantages

- Inexpensive
- Have a greater capacity than autoclaves
- The instruments are dry at the end of the cycle

Disadvantages

- Cannot be used for sterilization of handpieces
- Causes charring of some textiles
- Requires a much longer sterilization time than does autoclaving

Hot-air ovens are thus *not* ideal for the sterilization of dental instruments. Moreover few of the currently available models meet the requirement for an uninterrupted holding time of 60 minutes at 160 °C/320 °F.

Whatever method is used, it must be stressed that adequate time must be allowed for heating up and cooling down. Both are affected by size and number of instruments and by the way that they are loaded.

Monitoring of sterilization by autoclave or dry heat

In order to ensure that correct sterilizing conditions are being achieved, every process must be monitored regularly using sterilization-control indicators. These change colour when correct conditions have been attained and maintained for the correct length of time. The most widely used and therefore the most practical for general dentists are of two types: TST strips and Browne tubes.

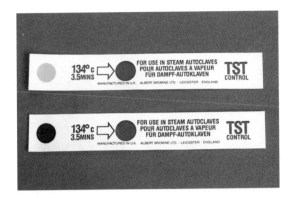

Figure 12.2

Time–steam–temperature strips: (a) before autoclaving;
(b) after autoclaving. The yellow disc on the left has
correctly turned purple.

Time–steam temperature strips

These are chemically coated, laminated strips which
change colour abruptly from yellow to blue–purple
when they have been subjected to the correct
heat–time ratio in saturated steam (Figure 12.2). If
any of the three criteria is not met, the indicators
do not change colour. There are two types
currently available. One type changes colour at
134 °C/273.2 °F after 3.5 minutes; the other, at
120 °C/248 °F after 15 minutes.

Browne tubes

These are glass tubes filled with fluid. They give
immediate visual indication by a colour change from
red to amber to green when the correct temperature to kill bacteria and spores has been attained.
They are principally for use in dry-heat sterilizers
but can also be used in autoclaves. However, they
are less convenient to use in the latter than TST
strips.

There are two types of tube available, one
changing colour after 1 hour at 150 °C/303 °F, the
other after 12 minutes at 180 °C/356 °F.

If either the TST strip or the Browne tube has not
turned to the correct colour after the sterilizing
process, that process must be considered suspect
and should be repeated using a fresh strip or tube.
Subsequent failures would indicate that the sterilization machine itself is at fault and must be
investigated.

Spore strips

These are paper strips impregnated with *Bacillus
stearothermophilus*, a spore-forming bacterium. The
strips are put in the densest part of the load, cycled
and then cultured afterwards. Any growth is
indicative of failure of sterilization.

In-dwelling thermocouples

These are placed in the chamber and accurately
monitor the temperature of sterilization. Provided
they are carefully calibrated, they are very accurate.

Chemical sterilization

Some chemical solutions can be used to sterilize
instruments, provided the instruments are soaked
in the solution at 20 °C/68 °F for 10 hours at the
concentration recommended by the manufacturer.
This is not always practicable and chemical sterilization is best reserved for those instruments for
which other methods are unsuitable. It is extremely
important that the instruments are thoroughly
cleaned first. Care must be taken to use only those
chemical sterilizing agents approved by the United
States Environmental Protection Agency. However, it must be stressed that there is no substitute
for autoclaving to obtain perfect sterility and
maintain the correct level of infection control.
Most chemical agents when suitably diluted are
best employed as antiseptic agents for chemical
disinfection.

Chemical disinfection

Many chemicals do not produce complete sterility since they do not destroy spores or some vegetative bacteria. They should primarily be used as disinfecting agents (primarily as hard-surface disinfectants), and also as holding solutions prior to sterilization. Waiting time prior to scrubbing can be used to soak instruments in a disinfecting solution. This keeps the organic material moist for easy removal and prevents spread of contaminants to other surfaces.

Ideal properties

- Provide rapid disinfection
- Have a broad-spectrum biocidal action
- Leave an anti-bacterial residue for continued biocidal activity
- Non-irritant to tissues of both dentist and patient
- Economical and with a re-use life of at least 21 days when diluted
- Complicated diluting procedures not required
- Change colour to show when it becomes non-active
- Contain a detergent to break up debris and contaminants
- Contain an anti-corrosion agent for protection of instruments
- Have Environmental Protection Agency approval

Gluteraldehyde

Gluteraldehyde is one of the most widely used solutions. Its effectiveness increases as pH increases and is greatest in an alkaline environment. However, when alkaline, gluteraldehyde tends to combine chemically with itself, forming polymers which are not biocidal. Stabilizing chemicals help to prevent this by allowing maximum activity without promoting polymerization. A neutral or alkaline solution is also less corrosive than an acid one.

Gluteraldehyde is usually used as a 2 per cent (w/v) solution, which rapidly destroys both vegetative and sporing bacteria.

Advantages

- Rapid action
- A wide range of biocidal activity on viruses and bacteria
- Non-corrosive
- Usable with plastic, rubber and heat-sensitive materials

Disadvantages

- Limited shelf-life
- Can irritate eyes and skin
- Can temporarily discolour the hands
- Requires the use of protective eyewear and gloves
- Some states in the USA have banned gluteraldehyde because it is carcinogenic in animals

Phenols

Since the first ones were widely used by Lister in 1867, new synthetically improved phenols have been created—mainly by combining chemicals with them which have synergistic properties.

Advantages

- Rapid and broad biocidal action
- Leave no residue
- Economical—when diluted 1 : 32 are effective for 60 days if unused
- Do not yellow the skin and are less toxic than gluteraldehyde.

Disadvantages

- Inactive against spores
- Some are ineffective against some bacteria and HBV

The most widely available for use in dentistry are biphenols, the best known of which is probably chlorhexidine, which is widely used for skin disinfection. Combined with 70 per cent alcohol, it is also an effective and economical hard-surface disinfectant.

Chlorhexidine has an additional advantage. It has been shown that in subcidal concentrations it diminishes the pathogenicity of bacteria (Holloway, Bucknell and Denton, 1986).

Diphenylalkane compounds are highly bactericidal. One of the commonest is hexachlorophene, which is an excellent skin disinfectant when made up in a 2–3 per cent concentration in the form of a cream or soap.

Alcohols

These are germicidal only when diluted. For rapid disinfection of the skin, 70 per cent isopropyl alcohol is useful. Alcohols are most commonly used in dentistry in combination with chlorhexidine as hand or hard-surface disinfectants. Wipes impregnated with alcohol and ethanol are available for use as small-surface disinfectants.

Halogens

Those most commonly used are chlorine, used as sodium hypochlorite, and iodine.

Advantages

- In a 1 per cent (w/v) solution they are both active against most bacteria and viruses
- A 1 per cent solution of iodine in alcohol is effective against some fungi and spores as well
- Leave a residue

Disadvantages

- Discolouration of hands and surfaces
- With the exception of sodium hypochlorite, the halogens cannot be used for sterilization

Iodophores

These are a combination of iodine and other organic compounds in a complex which releases iodine in small increments. This slow release provides continuous action, which can be monitored by the colour of the solution. When the amber colour changes to pale yellow, the solution should be changed. Iodophores are available in two forms:

- Surgical scrubs designed for use on skin and tissue but inappropriate for use as hard-surface disinfectant.
- Hard-surface disinfectants, which cannot be used on skin.

Both types must be used only as directed by the manufacturer and must always be diluted with water. It has been shown that the most effective dilution for use as a hard-surface disinfectant is 1:213 parts of water—they are more effective *diluted* than in concentrated form. One study (Molinari, Gleason, Cottore et al, 1987) has shown that, as surface disinfectants, properly diluted iodophore and sodium hypochlorite preparations are superior to 70 per cent isopropyl alcohol.

Advantages

- Broad biocidal action
- Leave a residue
- The surfactant carrier keeps the surface moist and residual action continues for some time after the surface appears to be dry
- Non-irritant to tissues
- Extremely economical
- Have a colour indicator

Disadvantage

- The iodine may discolour some surfaces and the hands when applied continuously over a period of time.

Quaternary ammonium compounds

When used alone, these have a low biocidal activity and do not kill spores or HBV. At a dilution of

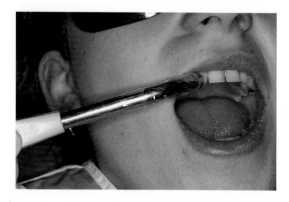

Figure 12.3

Plastic film has been wrapped around the rod of the curing light.

1 : 750 in 70 per cent ethanol they reduce the numbers of micro-organisms on hard surfaces and also leave a residue on evaporation of the alcohol. However, some authorities do not believe they should be used alone because of their low biocidal activity, and they are classified by the American Dental Association as 'not acceptable' as a disinfectant or sterilization agent.

Sterilization of connected instruments

Handpieces

Handpieces are one of the principal sources of cross-infection, since all types of handpiece are often contaminated with blood and saliva during cavity and crown preparations and prophylaxis. It is now possible to obtain autoclavable, high-speed handpieces as well as contra-angle and prophylaxis heads with quick-release couplings. A minimum

number of three of each type of handpiece should be in every treatment area to facilitate autoclaving between each patient.

Air–water syringes

These can now be obtained with removable nozzles and, like handpieces, a minimum of three per treatment area is essential, so that they can be autoclaved between patients. Where only a single handpiece or syringe tip is available, these must be thoroughly disinfected between every patient.

Visible and light curing tips

Contamination of that part of the tip placed intra-orally can be greatly reduced by wrapping transparent cling-film around the tip and handle (Figure 12.3) so that this is completely protected from contamination while allowing the light to penetrate. The intensity of the light emitted is probably reduced by no more than 3 per cent. They are in any event much less likely to become contaminated with blood and it is considered that this method, together with chemical disinfection, is adequate to prevent cross-infection.

Cross-infection control for impressions and appliances

Some potential infectious agents can survive outside the infected person's body, on prostheses, impressions, bite registrations and casts (Blakeslee and Wolff, 1988). This means that laboratory technicians could be exposed to infective organisms and steps must be taken to eliminate this risk.

In the dental practice

The recommended clinical procedure for control of cross-infection for impressions is first to rinse the impression to remove saliva, blood and debris.

The importance of rinsing cannot be over-emphasized, since it dilutes the concentration of micro-organisms to a level below the probable minimum infection dose. The impression should then be disinfected (ADA Council on Dental Materials, Dental Practice and Therapeutics, 1988). The method of disinfection depends on the impression material used. Alginate impressions can be coated with a disinfectant that has been accepted for use as a surface disinfectant and then sealed in a plastic bag prior to despatch to the dental laboratory. If the model is to be cast in the practice, it should be sealed first in the plastic bag for the recommended disinfection time before casting.

Polysulfide and addition silicone impression materials can be disinfected by immersion in any of the products accepted by the American Dental Association. Polyether impression materials may be adversely affected with disinfection by immersion. A chlorine compound with short disinfection time or a spray should be used (ADA Council on Dental Materials, Dental Practice and Therapeutics, 1988). There is no information available on the successful disinfection of hydrocolloid impressions.

In the dental laboratory

A 'chain of infection' extends through the laboratory (Blakeslee and Wolff, 1988). Incoming impression or other lab work may be contaminated with bacteria which then infect other laboratory areas, such as lab pans, pumice wheels, curing pots and burs. These, in turn, may infect cases which are being processed in the laboratory and the infection is thus passed onto another patient.

In addition, the technician is placed at risk from the handling of these appliances. It is possible to be cut with laboratory instruments, thus directly transmitting bacteria into the bloodstream. A strict protocol is therefore necessary for the dental laboratory.

Precautions which should be taken within the laboratory include the following:

- All work surfaces should be kept clean and disinfected regularly
- Periodic sterilization of all hand instruments and burs

- All case pans should be wiped prior to despatch from the laboratory
- All polishing wheels should be disinfected daily (or sterilized, if gas sterilization is available)
- All pumice pans should be changed daily
- Effective splash-guards should be used wherever applicable
- Water impression curing pots and heat curing units should be changed daily

Sterilization

The conventional sterilizing methods used in the dental treatment area cannot be used in the dental laboratory. Gluteraldehyde solution is absorbed by dental stone, plastics and rubbers, while iodophor and chlorine solutions are inconvenient to use because of the difficulty in controlling vapours and the stains produced. Heat sterilization cannot be used because the high temperatures required result in stone models crumbling, plastics distorting and impression material losing accuracy.

Gas sterilization is the only suitable method of sterilization for the dental laboratory. However, in general, it is not economically viable for dental practices or laboratories to possess a gas sterilizer and, in practical terms, good disinfection is adequate.

Receiving area

A receiving area should be established which is separate from the production area. Non-sterilized cases should not be taken beyond this area. It should be equipped with a smooth unseamed countertop, sink, stone bin and model vibrator. Workers in the area should wear a full length lab coat, protective glasses and latex gloves.

Unless the laboratory knows that the incoming work has been disinfected by the dental practice, all cases should be cleaned and disinfected as they are received. Where gas sterilization is available, impressions can be rinsed and then immediately poured. When set, the models can be separated, wrapped and placed in a gas sterilizer.

Production area

The production area should be kept entirely separate from the receiving area. Work surfaces and equipment should be kept free from debris and disinfected daily.

Despatching area

Outgoing models and prosthetic stages should be disinfected or sterilized if possible before they are returned to the dental practice. If gas sterilization is used, care must be taken for any appliance to be immediately air washed to prevent the danger of tissue irritation from the ethylene dioxide.

Clothing

One of the strange inconsistencies in dental practice is that though most dentists pay great attention to hygiene and sterilization of the practice itself, there are still a great many who work in their outdoor clothes with merely a short dental coat over the upper half of their body. Dirt and organisms from the street are thus brought into the treatment area and are a possible source of contamination. Also contaminants can be carried to the dentist's own home by clothes worn in the treatment area.

With the wide range of smart, inexpensive dental uniforms available today, there is no excuse for such an economy and, before commencing work in the morning, every dentist and DA should completely change into a clean working uniform, including top, trousers, socks and shoes. Coats and smocks should be preferably short sleeved since long sleeves can pick up debris and bacteria because they are nearer the mouth. Bare arms can be scrubbed in a suitable bactericidal skin cleanser.

Working in a clean uniform is not only a matter of basic hygiene but looks much more correct and conveys the right professional image to the patient.

Infection control protocols are constantly being updated. In addition, materials and techniques are continually being developed. For these reasons, the general practitioner must keep up-to-date with the latest guidelines issued by relevant government agencies, as well as with information available in professional journals and at trade exhibitions.

13 Work simplification and systems

Work simplification has been defined as 'the shortest and easiest way to practise dentistry' (Kilpatrick, 1979) and as 'minimizing the number of variables, so permitting the dental team to function more effectively' (Stombaugh, 1979). It may involve the rearrangement of equipment, instruments and materials in order to place them in a more favourable relationship to the team and a replanning of procedures.

Any attempt to achieve improvement in practice efficiency must involve a high degree of work simplification.

Advantages

- Reduces decision-making
- Improves speed and efficiency: 'Work becomes easier and is therefore accomplished in a shorter period of time' (Kilpatrick, 1979)
- Reduces optical fatigue
- Reduces stress and tension
- Provides a more relaxed working environment
- Produces a higher standard of work

Though much work simplification can be achieved by the application of common sense, its effectiveness can be greatly increased by adhering to some basic guiding principles.

Principles

Planning

Tray settings, and the choice of instruments to be included on them, should be based on the normal sequence of instrument use for each procedure. Such a sequence will depend on each dentist's personal preference. All instruments used only infrequently should be housed separately from the standard setting. Over-stocking trays produces overcrowding and is to be avoided since this defeats the purpose of the system. Multi-purpose tray settings should be avoided for the same reason.

Minimum numbers

Determination of the minimum number of instruments involves the following stages:

- For each procedure, the DA must list which instruments are used most frequently and which are not used routinely
- From the list, the dentist must then choose what he believes to be the correct set of instruments for every procedure
- The dentist must then closely question the need for having all the instruments chosen on every standard tray setting for each procedure and try to eliminate as many as possible
- Double-ended instruments should be used wherever possible and instruments chosen which can be used for several tasks

It will usually be found that many supposedly essential instruments are in fact used very infrequently and these should therefore be eliminated from the standard tray setting. Instruments used only occasionally can be placed on subsidiary trays or in drawers easily accessible to the dentist or DA. Such instruments would then have to be verbally requested by the dentist as they are not in the standard sequence. By minimizing the

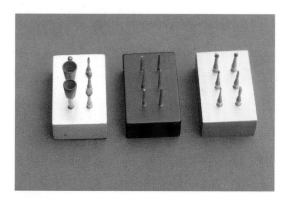

Figure 13.1

Colour-coded bur blocks containing burs required for different operations. From left to right, those shown are for polishing restorations, crown preparation and cavity refining.

Standardization

Every dentist is an individual and therefore each will perform the same task in different ways and with different instruments. It is important for each dentist to analyze which are his instruments of choice for each procedure and to determine the sequence in which he prefers to use them. Having made this decision, he should always employ the same sequence of instruments for the same procedure every time that procedure is carried out. Thus a rationalized work pattern is developed. In this way, the DA will be able to anticipate which instrument the dentist needs as treatment proceeds. Knowledge of both the steps in the procedures and the dentist's work pattern helps the DA to be more efficient and all operative procedures to be performed smoothly.

Anticipation

Anticipation is the key to work simplification, smooth working and good team dentistry. Ideally, the DA should know which instrument or material is required just *before* the dentist actually requires it.

number of instruments, 'hunt and search time' is reduced and the DA can choose the next instrument in a sequence more quickly.

This principle should also be extended to burs, which should be reduced to the minimum number needed for each type of procedure and placed in colour-coded bur blocks. It is important that very small blocks are used, since larger blocks tend to obey 'Parkinson's law'—that is, they get filled in proportion to the number of spaces available. Blocks should be of the exact size, to contain no more than the precise number of burs necessary for the procedure. For example there should be an individual bur block for high-speed burs for routine restorative procedures, crown preparation, cavity refining and polishing restorations. The blocks must be of an autoclavable material such as metal and ideally of different colours to allow colour coding (Figure 13.1).

Utilization

To help minimize frequent instrument transfer and achieve a smoothly flowing working sequence, every instrument should be used until its work is finished before moving to the next one in the sequence.

Correct location

It is surprising to find that a very high percentage of dentists still keep all hand instruments on their working side. This means that the dentist and not the DA picks up and replaces the instruments. This totally precludes the use of four-handed dentistry since it makes a full exchange system impossible.

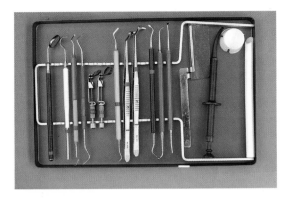

Figure 13.2

A pre-set tray for an amalgam restoration. The colour of the tray indicates that it is set for amalgam procedures. Each type of instrument has a different coloured sleeve on its shaft. The single narrow blue band on all the instruments denotes that they belong to an amalgam tray from treatment area No. 1. Together the bands form a diagonal line. The single white band on the tray shows that it belongs to treatment area No. 1.

All unnecessary movement and breaks in concentration can be eliminated by locating all instruments and materials on the DA's working side and by using her to pass and exchange them (see Chapter 11).

Location of materials should be based on their frequency of use. Those most frequently used are placed nearer to the DA than those used less frequently. Because of the increase in the range of materials now being used in general practice, it has to be accepted that some will have to be housed in locations away from the immediate chairside working surface and storage drawers. This should be minimized by providing more cupboard space as near to the chairside as possible. This should be located above worktop height, preferably within arm's reach of the DA to eliminate bending and over-stretching. The situation can be further improved by keeping to a minimum the amount of materials stored in the treatment area itself. It is acceptable for the dentist to change burs himself since this can often be quicker and more efficient. In this case, the bur block would be located on the dentist's working side, one of the few exceptions to the rule previously referred to. However, where the dentist prefers the DA to change burs, the bur block would remain on the DA's side.

Tray systems

One of the essential components of any work-simplification system is the use of pre-set trays for the instruments and materials required for each procedure. Such a tray should contain all such instruments and/or materials, arranged in correct sequence of use (Figure 13.2).

Advantages

● Change-over time is reduced because the used tray can be exchanged for a new one in a matter of seconds. The used tray can then be cleaned, sterilized and re-set by the member of staff responsible, who should preferably be a member of the clinical staff other than the chairside DA.
● The system allows unexpected and emergency procedures to be dealt with immediately. For example a dentist working on what was predicted to be a routine conservation procedure may find the pulp becomes exposed and requires root-canal therapy. This can be dealt with immediately since both the rubber-dam and endodontic trays are fully set and available for immediate use.
● The setting of a tray with standardized instruments in correct sequence of use is simplified and can be performed by junior or untrained members of staff.

Tray design

Trays should be made of metal (Figure 13.2) or of autoclavable plastic. They should be perforated if autoclaving is the method of sterilization, but can be solid if hot air is used. A tray should be large enough to contain all the instruments for a procedure and of correct size to fit into the autoclave. Use of trays made of non-autoclavable material would result in sterile instruments being placed on non-sterile trays, and this type is therefore not recommended unless used in conjunction with a sterile paper cover as described on page 138. All trays should have some means of keeping instruments in position: a shallow rack is suitable for metal trays; a moulded surface is required if plastic trays are employed.

Trays should be colour coded according to the type of procedure for which they are used. This can be achieved by using trays of different coloured materials. For example, all trays set for amalgam procedures would be the same colour; those for composite, examination and endodontic or crown and bridge procedures would be of different colours. Alternatively, if trays are of a uniform colour, autoclavable colour-coding tape can be applied to the tray. Whatever the colour-coding system used, a second colour should be added to denote the treatment area to which the tray belongs. This ensure that trays are returned to the correct area after sterilization. Colour coding can be done in one of two ways:

- Different numbers of stripes of the same colour can be used to denote the different treatment areas. Thus treatment area 1 would have one stripe on its trays, area 2, two stripes and so on (Figure 13.2).
- Alternatively each treatment area can be given a specific code colour and a single stripe of that colour placed on every tray belonging to it.

In order to avoid confusion, the stripe denoting type of procedure should be of a material noticeably wider than that designating treatment area. Vinyl electric tape is suitable for this purpose.

Tray storage

Tray racks should be used and these should be located *above* worktop height for ease of access by the DA. They should be either in front of her or to her right-hand side, and within arm's reach. The simplest type of rack consists merely of an open-fronted cabinet with wooden or metal runners to carry the trays.

Ideally there should be two racks, one for clean, sterilized trays and one for soiled trays which opens directly into the sterilization area. In this way, trays can be loaded onto the soiled tray rack immediately after use and then taken into the sterilization area by the second assistant for cleaning and sterilization. The sterile trays are then placed in the clean racks which pass directly into the treatment area.

Some autoclavable trays are too large to fit into the small autoclaves which are used in many general practices. In this case, the instruments have to be unloaded from the working tray, cleaned and then loaded into a small instrument basket or tray of correct size to fit the autoclave. The surface of working trays which cannot be autoclaved must be covered by a sterile disposable paper cover, with a new cover being provided for each occasion of use.

Planning a tray system

The decision on the number of each type of tray depends on several factors:

- The patient load per day for each treatment area.
- The frequency of each type of procedure. For example, a dental practice which predominantly deals with amalgam restorations would have a large number of amalgam trays, whereas one in which crown and bridge procedures predominate would have very few amalgam trays, but a large number of crown and bridge ones. Examination and X-ray trays are usually the most numerous but, because of the small number of instruments, much smaller trays can be used and these also have the advantage of fitting directly into even the smallest autoclave.
- The sterilization (dead) time required.

An emergency tray, pre-sterilized and pre-packed for oral surgery procedures, should always be available because, if for example a root is accidentally fractured during a routine extraction, the tray can be immediately brought into use to perform a surgical removal of the root. Similarly the endodontic tray should always be on hand for restorative procedures in case pulp exposure should occur.

The tub-tray system

This is a refinement of the tray system. It comprises two sections—a normal, flat tray on which the instruments are placed and a second, deeper tray of corresponding colour on which are placed all the relevant materials, mixing pads and spatulas. The second tray does not require autoclaving since no instruments are placed on it.

Because tubes and boxes of impression materials are so space-consuming, they have to be stored in cupboards or deep drawers. Of necessity, such storage spaces are further away from the DA's immediate work surface than are the instrument drawers, and so entail movement away from the immediate chairside. The tub-tray system precludes the need for this.

A modification of the normal work station to provide deeper rack storage allows the tubs containing the materials to be stored together with the instrument trays at the chairside. Alternatively specifically designed mobile carts are obtainable, which provide a well into which the tub and tray fit.

Setting a tray

- Collect all standardized instruments together.
- Ensure each instrument is placed in correct sequence of use.
- Keep instruments sterile until ready for use by employing a tray lid or cover.

Initially every standard tray setting should be photographed. The photographs should then be posted up in the room in which the trays are sterilized and re-set. This enables the trays to be set very accurately and quickly. Photographs are particularly useful when training junior members of staff, who will almost immediately be able to set the trays easily and correctly.

Colour coding

Identification of instruments by colour rather than shape is quicker, easier and less fatigue-producing because it reduces 'hunt and search' time.

Tray coding

Trays are coloured according to the type of procedure for which they are required. In a multi-operator practice, all trays should have a second colour-code stripe (or stripes) to denote the treatment area to which they belong, as described earlier in this chapter (see Figure 13.2).

Instrument coding

Every hand instrument should be coded with a colour specific to the type of instrument. Thus all instruments of the same type should have the same coloured sleeve (see Figure 13.3). A second, narrower band of colour should be used to denote the tray to which it belongs. These narrow bands should be placed on the shafts in such a location that when the instruments are laid in correct sequence of use on the tray, these bands form a diagonal line (see Figure 13.2). This ensures that when setting the tray the instruments are placed in correct sequence and also that when the tray is in use, the DA replaces each used instrument back in its correct position.

In a large practice, the number of these narrow stripes can be varied to correspond to the number of the treatment area to which the instrument belongs (Figure 13.3). This facilitates its return to the correct area after sterilization.

Rotary instruments

Either self-coloured blocks for burs or standard blocks with coloured tape or paint should be used, as described on page 150.

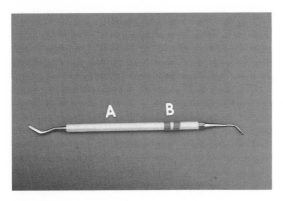

Figure 13.3

Instrument coding showing the bands denoting type of instrument (A) and tray type and treatment area number (B). This instrument is from an amalgam tray belonging to treatment area 2, denoted by the two bands.

Materials for colour coding

All materials should be autoclavable.

Coloured varnish

This can be painted on the instrument and baked for 6 hours at 200 °C/392 °F.

Heat-shrunk tubing

This is polythene tubing supplied in five colours. It can be cut to size, placed on the instrument shaft as a loose fit and will shrink tightly onto the instrument when placed in a hot oven for 5 minutes. It can be cut to any length and is therefore suitable to use for all coding functions.

Adhesive tape

This is supplied in several colours and is used by wrapping it around the instrument shaft and sealing the end.

Silicone rubber

This is supplied as narrow rings which are simply stretched onto the instrument shaft. Their main disadvantage is that, in view of their very narrow width, several rings of the same colour have to be placed together on the shaft if the instrument typing is to be clearly defined, as shown in Figure 13.3.

Part III   Applications to clinical procedures

14 Preparatory procedures

Rubber dam

The use of rubber dam in general practice is becoming increasingly important. In addition to its use in endodontics, the advent of techniques involving bonding of materials to enamel and dentine has required isolation from moisture which can only be perfectly achieved by using rubber dam. Thus anterior and posterior composites, adhesive bridges and splints, porcelain veneers and inlays all require the strict isolation from moisture contamination that only rubber dam can provide.

Major objections advanced by those dentists who still refuse to use rubber dam are that it is difficult to apply and very time-consuming. However, these problems often arise because the dentists have lost the skills learned as students through lack of routine use of rubber dam in general practice. A well-organized system and good team dentistry will overcome both these objections, help the dentist to apply rubber dam both easily and quickly, and thereby ensure its use wherever necessary.

Equipment required

Rubber dam

Heavy-duty dam in 13 cm or 15.5 cm squares should be used. The use of heavy-duty material precludes the possibility of it splitting and tearing and so makes placement extremely easy.

Stamp

This provides a series of dots representing all the teeth in the upper and lower arches, with lines marking the centre line, cuspids and first molars in each arch. By using it with an inking pad, many sheets of dam can be pre-stamped with this diagram. It therefore provides clear and easy reference points for the DA to punch the necessary holes for each case prior to the patient being seated. Indeed, quick reference to the case notes will often show the DA precisely which teeth are to be isolated.

Rubber-dam punch

This should be capable of cleanly punching holes of varying diameters.

Rubber-dam clamps

A minimum number should be selected which will give sufficient choice for use on both anterior and posterior teeth. Such a selection might comprise Nos 00, 2, 7, 8, 8A, 9 and 14. This may be varied by individual preference, but the number must be kept small to minimize 'hunt and search' time. The clamps should be kept in an organizer box (Figure 14.1), or a clamp-holding rack, for ease of selection.

Rubber-dam clamp holder

This must grip the clamp holes firmly yet be easy to disengage from the clamp after it has been placed if it is not to pull the clamp off the tooth.

Rubber-dam frame

This can be of metal or plastic and is either U- or oval-shaped with cleats or sharp spikes on which the free end of the dam can be hooked.

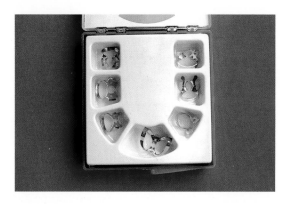

Figure 14.1

A basic selection of rubber-dam clamps in a colour-coded organizer box.

Other items

Other items which are helpful, though not essential, include a probe or flat plastic instrument for everting rubber-dam material over the edges of the gingivae, a tube of shaving cream to lubricate the dam surface and facilitate its placement, and floss ligatures which may be sometimes used in place of a clamp. Rubber-dam napkins of absorbent paper can be placed under the dam to separate it from the patient's face and absorb moisture, so providing greater comfort.

Pre-preparation

A pre-set tray or trays must be prepared which should contain all the instruments and materials required. By having all the necessary instruments collected together and readily to hand, the placement of rubber dam becomes far easier and quicker. The dentist will thus be more inclined to use it routinely—to the advantage of himself and the patient through the improvement in the standard of his work.

Clinical procedure

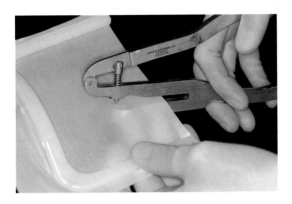

Figure 14.2

Having stretched the rubber-dam square over the frame and engaged it securely on the retaining spikes, the DA punches holes in the dam in the area specified by the dentist. In general three holes are punched—one for the tooth being treated and one each for the tooth mesial and the tooth distal to it.

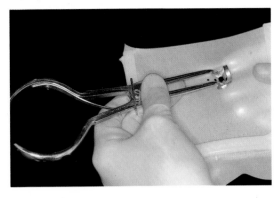

Figure 14.4

The DA holds the forceps by their beaks in her left hand in a palm grip, supporting the clamp and rubber dam with her right hand palm upwards underneath them.

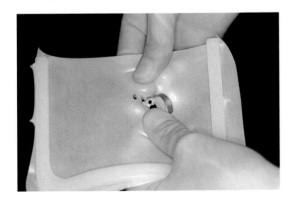

Figure 14.3

The DA selects the correct clamp, inserts the clamp into the most distal hole punched in the dam and loads it into the clamp forceps.

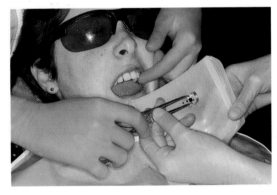

Figure 14.5

The DA presents the forceps, clamp and dam to the dentist into his palm grasp as he retracts the patient's lip with his left index finger. The dentist firmly grasps the clamp forceps and the DA releases her left hand while still supporting the dam with her right.

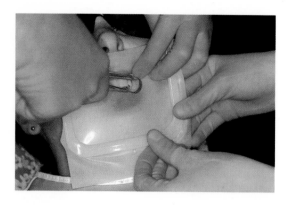

Figure 14.6

The dentist places the clamp over the tooth while the DA maintains a grasp of the corners of the dam frame nearest to her.

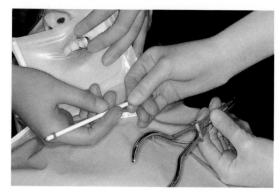

Figure 14.8

Having taken away the clamp forceps, the DA directly places the probe into the dentist's pen grasp using her right hand.

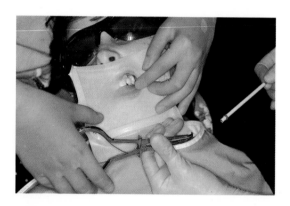

Figure 14.7

Having placed the clamp firmly on the tooth, the dentist disengages the forceps. The DA then takes the forceps from him with her left hand while holding a plastic instrument or probe ready in her right hand.

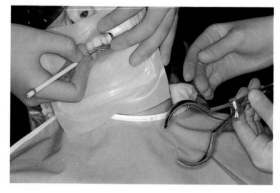

Figure 14.9

The dentist uses the probe to evert the edges of the dam around the gingival margin while the DA maintains her right hand near the border of the frame ready to receive the probe when the dentist has finished with it.

This is an excellent example of the use of four hands simplifying a procedure which might otherwise be extremely difficult.

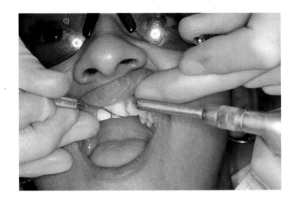

Figure 14.10

Examination. The DA dries the tooth and gingivae while the dentist uses the probe.

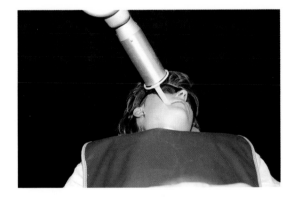

Figure 14.11

A bite-wing X-ray photograph being taken of the patient's right upper and lower lower quadrants. Her head has been rotated 45° to her left.

Examination and X-rays

Multiple pre-set trays must be prepared. These can be smaller than those required for other procedures. They should contain a mirror, sickle and interproximal probes, pocket measuring probe, two X-ray films, either mounted in a holder or with bite-wing tabs attached, and an X-ray envelope.

Clinical procedure

The DA passes the mirror and probe by direct placement. The technique is fully described on page 121.

At all times while the dentist is performing the intra-oral examination, the DA must keep the teeth and soft tissues dry by using an air–water syringe and following the point of the dentist's probe as he moves it around the mouth (Figure 14.10). This procedure will ensure a much higher standard of diagnosis since a dry tooth surface shows lesions more readily than one covered with saliva. A dry mucosa and gingival margin also gives a more accurate indication of periodontal health. The DA holds the syringe in her left hand, leaving her right hand free to chart on the record card.

X-ray procedure

Where an X-ray machine is available at the chairside, all intra-oral X-ray photographs can be taken with the patient placed in the fully supine position. There is absolutely no reason for the patient to be seated vertically during intra-oral X-ray.

Bite-wing X-rays

In order to ensure that the central ray passes exactly at right angles to the film, the patient's head should be rotated to the right when taking X-ray photographs of the left quadrants and to the left when taking the right quadrants (Figure 14.11).

Conventional syringe

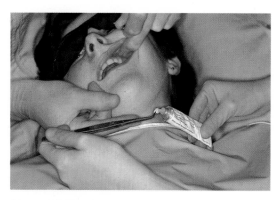

Figure 14.12

Surface anaesthesia: the DA places tweezers holding a cotton pledget coated with surface anaesthetic directly into the dentist's right hand.

These are precisely the same rotation movements as were described on page 80. In this way, the chair does not have to be raised vertically as high as it would if the head were kept vertical. However, there is a lower limit beyond which most X-ray machine arms will not go so that the chair will need to be raised vertically and to a height rather greater than it would be for restorative procedures.

Periapical X-rays

In addition to rotating the patient's head, as described for bite-wing X-rays, it may also need to be tilted forwards or backwards to facilitate the lining up of the central beam at right angles to the film if the holder is of the type which uses this technique, or at right angles to the line bisecting the angles, if the bisected angle technique is used.

Local anaesthesia

Surface anaesthesia

The DA prepares a cotton pledget in locking tweezers or a cotton bud and coats it in surface

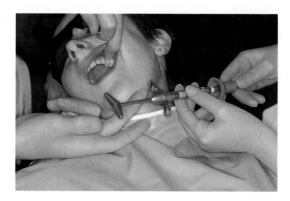

Figure 14.13

The syringe must at all times be kept out of the patient's view by presenting it in the transfer zone. This will ensure that it is outside the supine patient's range of peripheral vision and so will keep patient apprehension to a minimum.

The DA grasps the syringe, holding it between her left thumb and index finger, mid-way along the barrel. Her right hand holds the shaft of the finger-guard which is over the needle sheath. The DA directs the plunger towards the dentist, who has placed his right hand in the transfer zone, palm upwards, with his index and middle fingers parted about 3 cm and his thumb upright. The DA places the plunger into the angle between the dentist's thumb and index finger (or in contact with the pad of the thumb, depending on the preference of the dentist).

anaesthetic. This is directly placed into the dentist's right hand (Figure 14.12). Whilst he applies the anaesthetic, she flames the end of the cartridge and loads it into the hypodermic syringe.

Transferring the syringe

A two-handed placement technique must be used to preclude the possibility of the DA's hand contaminating the sterile needle (Figures 14.13–14.17). This technique allows the same syringe and needle to be used on the same patient, should a supplementary injection be required.

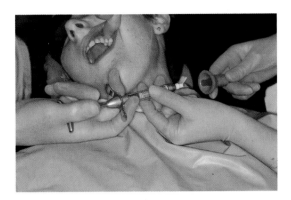

Figure 14.14

When the DA feels that the dentist has a firm grasp on the syringe, she removes her left hand from the barrel and at the same time pulls off the needle sheath with her right hand. Since her hand is moving away from the needle, this eliminates possible contact with it.

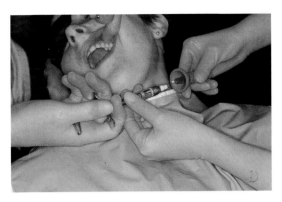

Figure 14.16

The DA takes back the syringe by grasping the barrel with her left hand and replacing the sheath onto the needle with her right.

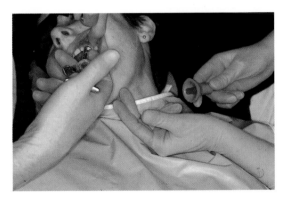

Figure 14.15

The DA must maintain her hands in this position while the dentist carries out the injection. This ensures that after the injection she is ready immediately to take back the syringe.

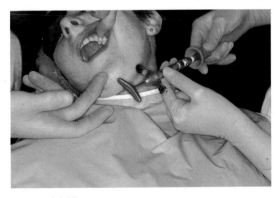

Figure 14.17

The dentist then releases his grasp and the syringe, with the sheath firmly in place over the needle, is removed by the DA. Resheathing the needle must only be performed with a finger-guard firmly placed over the needle sheath to avoid the danger of needle stab injury.

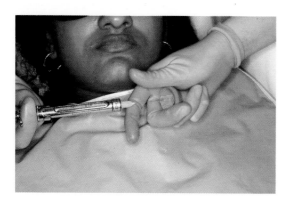

Figure 14.18

A one-handed syringe transfer showing the needle moving across the DA's fingers.

It should be noted that if the DA were to use a one-handed transfer, the needle sheath could only be removed by her moving her hand along the barrel and onto the sheath. In pulling the sheath off, it would be extremely easy for the DA to touch the needle with the palm of her hand and so contaminate it (Figure 14.18).

After the patient has been dismissed, the used needle should be unscrewed from the syringe by holding the barrel portion of the finger-guard and placing the sharp end of the needle into the 'sharps' box. The needle and the sheath can be ejected into it without any possibility of touching the needle. If, however, the dentist prefers not to resheath the needle but to dispose of it immediately, the DA must not take back the syringe after the injection has been given. Instead the dentist should dispose of the used needle in an appropriate piece of apparatus, which should be placed on his own working surface.

Aspirating syringe

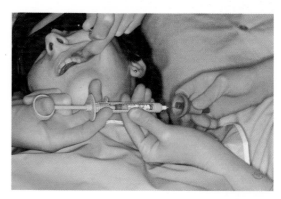

Figure 14.19

The DA must first check that the plunger has engaged the rubber piston in the cartridge by pulling it back. The method of presentation and placement is the same as for a conventional syringe, except that the ring of the plunger must not be placed between the dentist's thumb and index finger but carefully over his thumb, to allow him to withdraw the plunger when aspirating.

Intra-ligamentary syringe

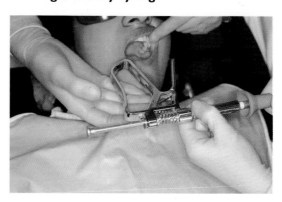

Figure 14.20

This is held by the dentist in a palm grasp and not a thumb/two-finger grasp. He must therefore hold out his hand with palm upwards and with fingers closed in the same position as if he were to receive any palm-grip instrument. The DA's grasp is virtually the same—her left hand is on the barrel and her right on the needle sheath. She then directly places the syringe into the dentist's open palm grasp.

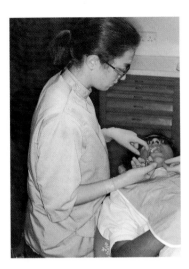

Figure 14.21: Upper right quadrant

Patient: Head rotated 15° to left (that is, away from the dentist), tilted backwards and with the mouth slightly closed to relax the cheek and lip.

Dentist: Location at 10 o'clock. The dentist is in perfect position with the upper arm vertical.

Injection techniques

Infiltration

The long axis of the needle must follow that of the tooth being anaesthetized. To achieve this while maintaining finger-control posture, the same principles must be followed as those for any operative procedure. The dentist should still maintain his frontal plane parallel to the tooth surface and his upper arm and elbow in contact with his body as described on pages 78–80. He must therefore use as many of the five variables as are necessary (Figure 14.21–14.22).

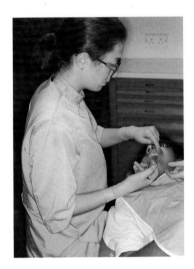

Figure 14.22: Upper left quadrant

Patient: As for the upper quadrant but with head rotated 45° to right (that is, towards the dentist).

Dentist: Location 10 o'clock. Perfect posture is maintained.

Nerve blocks

In most cases when giving the inferior dental block on the right side, it is not possible to maintain the elbow joint strictly in contact with the side of the body, so that some compromises to finger-control posture may have to be accepted, see Figures 14.23–14.24. The right inferior dental block is perhaps the most difficult injection to administer in the correct posture. However, it is worth noting that as the injection proceeds, the elbow naturally approximates towards the dentist's body. In addition, this procedure is a very short one so that any slight deviation from correct posture is only maintained for a few seconds.

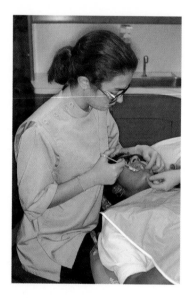

Figure 14.23: Inferior dental block—lower left

Patient: Head rotated 10° to the left with zero backwards tilt but with the mouth widely open.

Dentist: Location 9.30. Perfect posture is maintained.

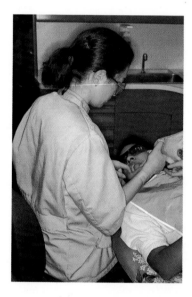

Figure 14.24: Inferior dental block—lower right

Patient: Head rotated 45° to the right with the head tilted forwards by the maximum amount possible and the mouth opened widely.

Dentist: Location 8.30. The upper arm is only very slightly abducted from the body, but otherwise the posture is good.

The direction of the needle is more in a vertical than horizontal direction for this nerve block.

Intra-ligamentary injection

The long axis of the needle must follow precisely the long axis of the tooth. Because the syringe is held in a palm grasp, it is more difficult to attain this than when using a conventional syringe. Even more careful attention must therefore be paid to the correct application of the five variables (see pages 78–80).

Failure to relate the needle to the long axis of the tooth correctly will cause considerable distortion of the dentist's right arm and shoulder and, as this injection needs to be given very slowly, this distortion will be maintained for a long period.

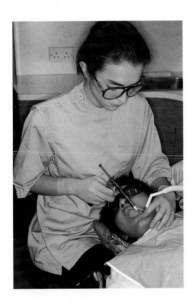

Figure 14.25: Mandibular quadrant

Patient: Head rotated 10° to the right or left depending on the quadrant being injected, tilted backwards and mouth widely open.

Dentist: Location 12 o'clock.

Maxillary quadrant

The variables are virtually identical to those previously given for administering of infiltrations with the conventional syringe.

15 Restorative procedures— amalgam

To demonstrate the application of the principles of team dentistry propounded in the previous chapters, the procedure involved in the restoration of a disto-occlusal cavity in an upper bicuspid will be described.

Local anaesthesia having been achieved, the dentist prepares the cavity using high-speed cutting. The DA maintains the aspirator on site to retract the patient's left lip and cheek. As the dentist is using reflected vision, the DA uses the air–water syringe to clear the pre-wetted mirror by dripping water intermittently onto its surface (see pages 112–13, Figure 10.15).

On completion of high-speed cutting, the dentist removes the caries using both spoon excavators and a slowly revolving rose-head bur. He may then wish to use fissure and end-cutting burs for final cavity-margin refinement. At this stage, the DA uses her air–water syringe to keep the cavity and mirror clear of debris, so providing unobscured vision for the dentist.

On completion of cavity preparation the DA mixes the lining material, taking care to mix near to the corner of the pad. While she is doing this, the dentist places a cotton roll in the sulcus and dries the cavity with *his* air–water syringe. If only one syringe is available, this will have been transferred to the DA's side (see page 105), and the dentist will have to use the DA's syringe to dry the cavity.

When she has finished mixing the lining material, the DA coats both ends of the placement instrument. She then places an excavator between her left ring and little fingers, the placement instrument between her left thumb and index finger, and the pad of lining material in her *right* hand. The corner of the pad bearing the lining material should be placed as near as possible to the patient's mouth and so within the field of the dentist's peripheral vision. The DA places the lining instrument directly into the dentist's right hand but retains the excavator in her little finger.

Clinical procedure

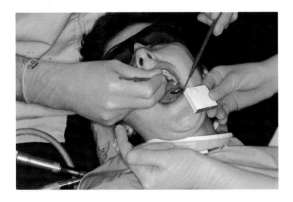

Figure 15.1

The dentist places the lining in position and, if necessary, scoops further quantities from the pad. Since the lining material on the pad is being held within his range of peripheral vision, the dentist is able to make minimal finger movements from the pad to the mouth without needing to take his eyes off the cavity. This helps to reduce fatigue from repeated re-accommodation.

While the lining is being placed, the DA holds her left thumb and index finger open ready to receive back the placement instrument by grasping it at its non-working end.

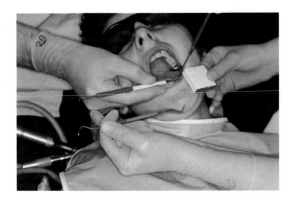

Figure 15.2

The DA removes the placement instrument and, using parallel exchange, places the excavator into the dentist's open fingers. He trims excess lining material from the cavity margin and finishes any necessary shaping with the excavator. While he is doing this, the DA turns to her working surface, discards the placement instrument and pad and picks up the appropriate matrix retainer and a flat plastic instrument.

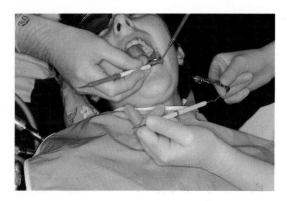

Figure 15.3

The DA turns towards the dentist holding the matrix at its working end between her right thumb and index finger and the flat plastic instrument (yellow) at its non-working end between her left thumb and index finger.

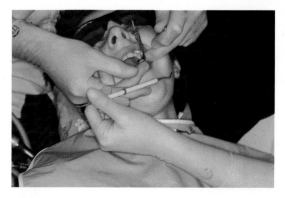

Figure 15.5

The dentist places the matrix band on the tooth and tightens the screw. The mirror is not needed at this stage and he can therefore rotate it backwards between his left thumb and index finger, tucking the shaft into his palm. This removes it from the operating site and allows free movement of his left middle and ring fingers to retract the lip while he tightens the matrix retainer and ensures that it does not trap the lip or soft tissue. Before the dentist completely tightens the matrix, the DA places the flat plastic instrument into the open fingers of his right hand.

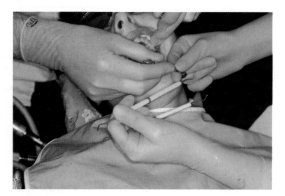

Figure 15.4

She moves the matrix retainer towards the dentist and places it directly into his right hand. She takes the excavator from the dentist, grasping it at its non-working end with her little finger, but maintains the plastic instrument in position in the transfer zone.

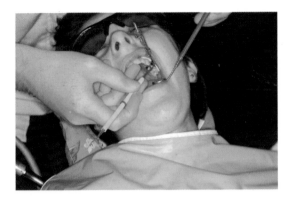

Figure 15.6

The flat plastic instrument is used to ensure that the band is seated properly over the gingival floor and also to burnish it in the contact area. While the dentist is completing band placement and burnishing, the DA picks up the wedge holder (in which a wedge has been pre-loaded), holding it at its non-working end in her left thumb and index finger.

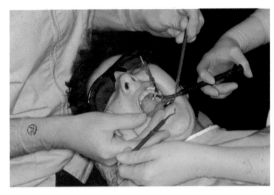

Figure 15.8

Next the DA mixes the amalgam, loads the carrier and picks up the first packing instrument at its non-working end between her left thumb and index finger. She places it into the dentist's right hand with the working end pointing upwards and immediately places the amalgam directly into the cavity, holding the amalgam carrier in her right hand. The dentist packs the amalgam. The DA loads the second carrier and repeats the procedure.

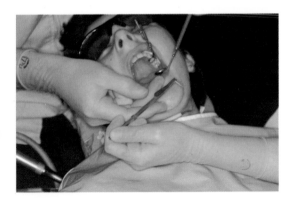

Figure 15.7

Using her left fifth finger, the DA removes the flat plastic instrument and, by parallel exchange, places the loaded wedge holder into the dentist's right hand. The dentist inserts the wedge. The DA maintains her left hand in position, with her thumb and index finger open ready to receive back the holder from the dentist. She then discards the holder and flat plastic instrument onto her work surface.

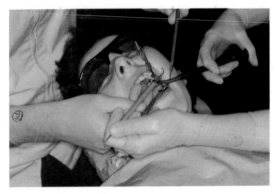

Figure 15.9

After the second placement of amalgam and before loading the carrier with a third increment, the DA picks up the second packer at its non-working end with her left hand, exchanges it for the first packer by parallel exchange and feeds the third increment of amalgam into the cavity. The procedure is then repeated until the dentist signals that he has sufficient amalgam.

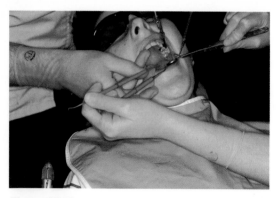

Figure 15.10

The DA discards the carrier and first packer and picks up a pair of dressing tweezers in her right hand and an amalgam carving instrument at its non-working end in her left. She removes the wedge with the tweezers and exchanges the second packer for the carving instrument into the dentist's right hand.

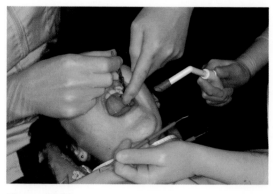

Figure 15.12

The DA removes the aspirator from the patient's mouth but retains it just outside the lips. She takes the carver from the dentist, but as the dentist will need to use it again immediately after removing the band, she retains it and the packer in the transfer zone.

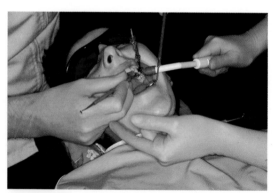

Figure 15.11

The DA discards the tweezers and wedge on her work surface and by a very small movement of her right hand picks up the aspirator tip, which she places 'on-site' but nearer to the tooth than she would for aspiration of fluid. She retains her left hand in position, holding the discarded packer in her left little finger, but with her thumb and index finger open while the dentist carves the gross excess from the marginal ridge of the restoration, *prior* to removal of the matrix. The aspirator tip is placed close to the site so that this initial piece of excess amalgam will go into the aspirator tube and not fall into the patient's mouth.

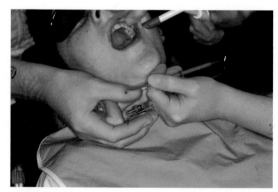

Figure 15.13

The dentist may now use both hands to remove the matrix, free it from the restoration and move it out of the mouth for the DA to grasp the working end between her middle and ring fingers.

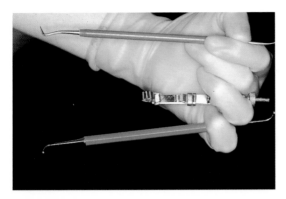

Figure 15.14

It is important to emphasize that at this stage both the discarded packer and the carver are still retained in their respective positions. The DA should *not* turn to her work surface to discard the instruments. Such a movement is unnecessary and would break the rhythm of the procedure. Thus the DA would be holding the carver between her thumb and index finger, the matrix retainer between her middle and ring fingers, and the packer between the ring and little fingers. In this way, the instruments are immediately available for the next stage.

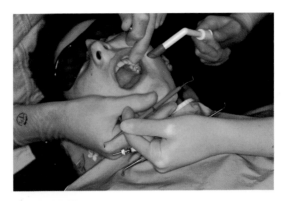

Figure 15.15

The DA places the carver directly into the dentist's right hand again.

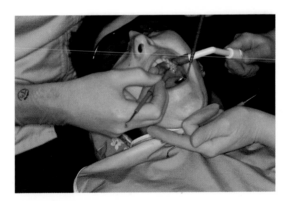

Figure 15.16

The dentist proceeds with occlusal carving and shaping of the restoration. The DA replaces the aspirator tip 'on site' as close as possible to the restoration to remove excess amalgam being carved from it.

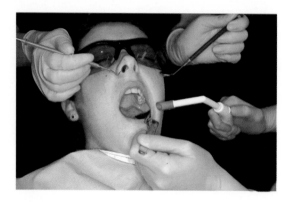

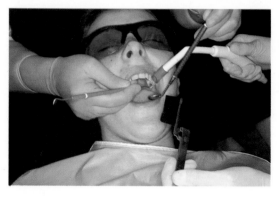

Figure 15.17

When the dentist has completed carving to his satisfaction, he still holds the mirror and carving instrument, but removes them from the mouth to indicate that the occlusion must be checked. Having set down the instruments held in her left hand, the DA picks up occlusal registration paper clamped in a suitable holder. The holder can be either one specifically made for the purpose or a pair of Spencer-Wells artery forceps.

The DA removes the aspirator from the mouth, places the paper over the restoration, requests the patient to close gently on it and then to open as widely as possible.

Figure 15.18

The DA removes the registration paper from the mouth but keeps it in the transfer zone ready for re-insertion. She replaces the aspirator tip on site and the dentist carves away any high spots which are marked.

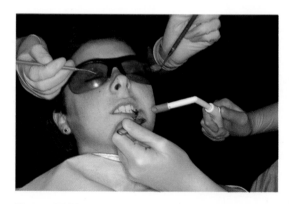

Figure 15.19

The DA once more removes the aspirator, the dentist removes the carver and mirror and the DA replaces the occlusal paper in the mouth, asking the patient to close once more. This sequence is repeated until the occlusion, both centric and excursive, is correct.

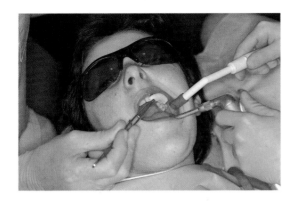

Figure 15.20

The DA washes the cotton roll prior to the dentist removing it with tweezers.

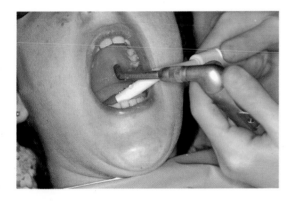

Figure 15.21

Before the patient sits up, the DA washes the palate and mouth, holding the aspirator in the Fauces position.

Patient dismissal

By the end of the procedure, the patient's mouth will have become very dry due to the continuous use of the aspirator during the final stages. This can have several consequences:

- The cotton roll can adhere to the sulcus and, if pulled off, may tear the mucosa
- Dried debris, such as excavated caries or pieces of amalgam carved from the restoration, adhere to the mucosa and tongue
- Pieces of carved amalgam lodge beneath the tongue
- The patient's mouth feels dry and unpleasant

Before the patient leaves the chair the DA must therefore:

- Retract the patient's lip with the aspirator and use her syringe to wet the cotton roll before the dentist removes it with tweezers (Figure 15.20)
- Use the air–water spray and aspirator together, systematically to wash around the mouth—the vigorous irrigation dislodges debris from the mucosa and pushes it posteriorly where it can easily be removed through the aspirator (Figure 15.21)
- Similarly wash in the sublingual area
- Wet the palate with a gentle spray of water

These procedures take only a few seconds and, since the mouth is wet and free of debris, the patient feels no desire to rinse. The DA then removes the patient's protective spectacles and bib and assists him off the chair and out of the treatment area.

Mouth rinsing

This traditional dental custom requires some rethinking in the light of the modern techniques now available, such as the one described above. Indeed the whole process of mouth rinsing is a most unhygienic and time-consuming process, which is to be discouraged as far as possible. Rinsing occurs both during treatment and at its completion. The former is often a ritual performed by the patient for purely psychological reasons, as a means of interrupting treatment. This is proved by the fact that the patient's desire to rinse occurs most frequently when the air turbine is being used, when the mouth is at its wettest and free of debris, and so at precisely the time the patient *least* needs to rinse.

The main disadvantage of intermittent rinsing while treatment is being delivered is that it disturbs the rhythm of work for the dentist and causes breaks in concentration. Moreover the movement to the spittoon invariably alters the patient's position in the chair. When rinsing is complete and the patient lies back again, his head is always replaced lower down the headrest, involving the need for the DA to reposition the patient again. These constant breaks and readjustments are extremely irritating and can be a major source of working stress.

Rinsing on completion of the procedure can be extremely time-wasting and places pressure on the dental team, particularly as they are trying to keep to a tight appointment schedule.

For all these reasons, whenever possible, use of the techniques described to eliminate rinsing is to be strongly recommended.

16 Restorative procedures— composites

Anterior composites

Preparation

Rubber dam and composite trays (Figure 16.1) should be made ready at the chairside. The latter should contain: etchant; resin bond; brushes which are clearly coded for etchant and bond placement; occlusal paper in a holder; two wedge holders loaded with wedges; suitable matrices and celluloid strips; blocks containing finishing burs and discs which should be mounted on mandrels in correct sequence of use; placement, packing and carving instruments specifically reserved for composite materials.

It is essential that these instruments should not be used with any other materials. They must therefore be specifically colour coded (Figure 16.1), in a way that clearly distinguishes them from instruments which have been used for other procedures and which would contaminate the composite materials.

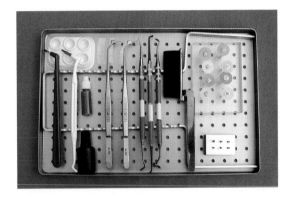

Figure 16.1

A pre-set tray for anterior composite restorations.

Clinical procedure

- Rubber dam should be placed in position and local anaesthetic administered, if required
- Aspiration and soft-tissue retraction techniques should be used as previously described
- Placement of lining: the technique is the same as that described for amalgam restoration, but smaller placement instruments are usually necessary—those with very small diameter ball ends are particularly useful

- The enamel is polished using oil-free pumice
- Etching and bonding: see Figures 16.2–16.6
- The DA discards the holder and dispenses a small amount of composite onto the corner of the pad
- She picks up the first placement instrument with her left hand, the pad with her right, turns to the dentist and, holding the pad near the patient's mouth, directly places the first packer into the dentist's hand

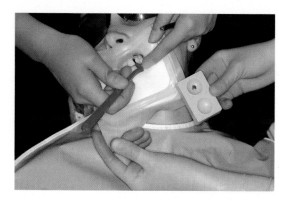

Figure 16.2

The DA loads the brush with etchant and, holding it at its end, directly places it into the dentist's pen grasp. While the dentist is painting the etchant onto the enamel, the DA holds her left hand in the transfer zone with index finger and thumb open ready to receive back the brush after the etchant has been applied.

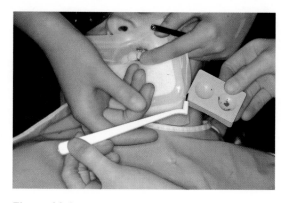

Figure 16.4

The DA loads the second brush with the bond and passes it by direct placement into the dentist's right hand. After the dentist has applied the bond, but prior to light curing it, the DA gently blows air onto the cavity and over the enamel surface to distribute the bond into a thin film and prevent accumulation of excess material.

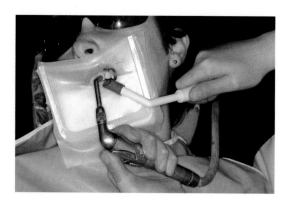

Figure 16.3

After the requisite time, the DA washes off the etchant, using the air–water syringe and aspirator on site and then thoroughly dries the cavity and margins.

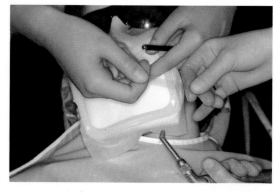

Figure 16.5

Still prior to curing, the DA passes a celluloid strip to the dentist and he places this between the cavity and the adjacent tooth to ensure that bond material is not retained by capillary action between the teeth. This is important, since bond cured between teeth prevents the future insertion of a strip.

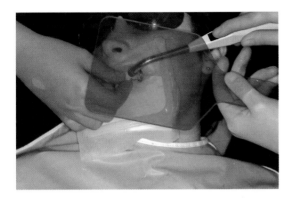

Figure 16.6

While the dentist holds the strip in place, the DA cures the bond, holding the light in her right hand and the cure shield over the patient's mouth in her left. This protects both the dentist and the DA from the glare of the curing light, and prevents retinal damage.

Placement of composite: The DA presents a pre-loaded wedge holder with her left hand, the dentist places the wedge and the DA removes the empty wedge holder. This procedure is identical to that described for amalgam restoration (see Figure 15.7).

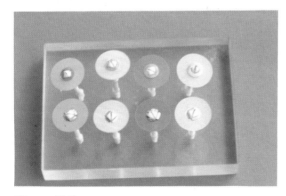

Figure 16.7

Finishing discs in sequence of use, pre-mounted on mandrels in a block.

- The dentist scoops a small quantity of composite and packs the first increment of material into the cavity.
  This stage and the two preceding it are similar to those described for placement of lining material (see Figures 15.1 and 15.2).
- Where composite is delivered using the gun and compule system, the DA should load the gun with a compule of the appropriate shade and place it into the dentist's palm grip.
- While the dentist holds the strip in place, the DA cures the first increment. Subsequent increments are placed and cured.
  This technique allows the dentist to have both hands free, which is often essential if strips and materials are to be held in the correct position, particularly when the cingulum area is being moulded.
- The DA removes the wedge with tweezers and receives the used strip from the dentist in her left hand.
- The rubber dam is removed.

Polishing

The dentist's preferred rotary finishing instruments should be arranged in a special block in sequence of use and kept to as small a number as possible. Discs should be pre-mounted on mandrels and also placed in a block in correct sequence of use (Figure 16.7).

Ideally, two rows of the complete disc sequence should be set out. One has the abrasive polishing side facing inwards (ie, towards the operator), and the other outwards (away from the operator). This eliminates the necessity for constant removal and reversal of discs.

Exchange of burs, discs or stones

When using rotary instruments, whether burs, discs or stones, in the slow-speed handpiece, the exchange will be much smoother and more rapid if a fully assisted technique is used (see Figures 16.8–16.11).

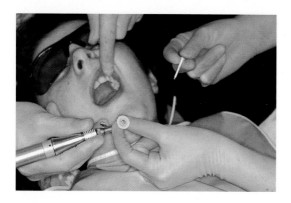

Figure 16.8

The dentist holds out the handpiece containing the used disc mandrel in the transfer zone. He releases the bur latch with his right index finger, maintaining it open whilst the DA removes the used mandrel with her left thumb and index finger.

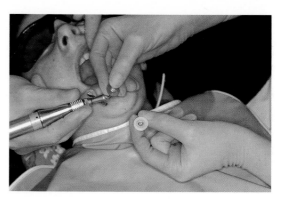

Figure 16.10

The DA places the second mandrel into the handpiece. When this is firmly in position, the dentist releases his index finger on the bur latch to lock in the new mandrel.

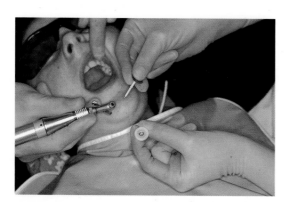

Figure 16.9

The dentist maintains his hand in the transfer zone. He keeps the latch open as the DA removes the first mandrel, while holding the second one ready in her right. She then moves the second one towards the handpiece.

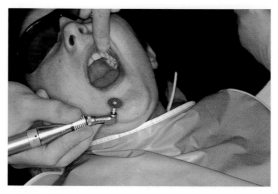

Figure 16.11

The dentist can then use the new mandrel immediately, while the DA makes ready the next disc. Subsequent discs are then sequentially removed and inserted.

If high-speed finishing burs are used, these must be changed by the dentist since the DA has both hands employed holding the aspirator and air–water syringe to retract tissue.

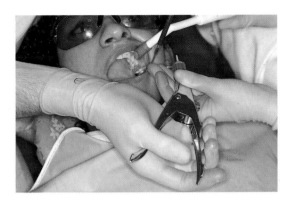

Figure 16.12

Capsulated glass-ionomer cement in the special syringe is placed by the DA into the dentist's reverse palm–thumb grasp by grasping it at its extreme end.

Glass-ionomer cements

These types of cement require very careful pro-portioning and mixing. They are available for either hand or automatic mixing.

Hand mixing

- The bottle must be shaken before dispensing the contents.
- The scraper at the mouth of the bottle must be used to ensure the correct amount of powder is dispensed.
- When the liquid is dispensed, the bottle must be held vertically.
- The powder must be drawn into the liquid and mixed very quickly (15 seconds maximum), using a small, flexible spatula.
- The surface of the mixed material must be shiny. If the surface appears dull, the material must be re-mixed before it is handed to the dentist.

- The technique of presentation, placement and exchange of material and instruments is the same as that described for amalgam or composite restorations.

Automatic mixing

The capsule must be pressed firmly for two full seconds, mixed automatically for the precise time recommended and loaded into the special gun provided. This is held at its extreme nozzle end and handed to the dentist in either palm or reverse palm–thumb grasp (Figure 16.12), depending on the location of the cavity.

Guidelines for use

Whether mixed by hand or automatically, these materials must be mixed and presented as rapidly as possible due to their short working time. Good four-handed technique is vital.

Before mixing is commenced, the cavity must be isolated and completely dry, and the dentist ready with his hand and fingers open in the transfer zone, ready to receive the material immediately it has been mixed. The DA should retract the lip and aspirate while the material is being placed.

One important addition to the procedure when using these materials is the need for immediate protection of the restoration or lining from moisture. Either a rapid drying varnish or a coating of light-cured, unfilled composite resin must there-fore be used.

Protection from moisture

In both the following techniques, the avoidance of any delay before a protective covering is applied precludes contamination from gingival seepage or other moisture.

Using varnish

While the dentist retains his grip on either the celluloid strip or cervical matrix, the DA dispenses a small quantity of varnish into the well of a suitable

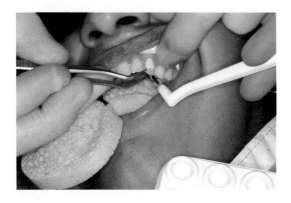

Figure 16.13

The dentist prepares to remove the cervical matrix from a glass–ionomer restoration on the upper canine. The DA holds the brush wetted with varnish very near to the tooth.

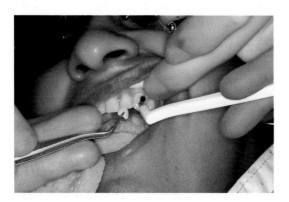

Figure 16.14

The dentist has completely removed the matrix and the DA immediately coats varnish onto the surface of the restoration.

container. She holds this in her left hand and the brush in her right, both as near to the mouth as possible. When the dentist signals he is ready to remove the matrix or strip, the DA coats the brush with varnish and holds it as near as possible to the restoration (Figure 16.13). As the matrix is removed she is thus able immediately to paint varnish over the surface of the cement (Figure 16.14).

Using composite resin

A similar procedure is used, except that the DA holds the brush loaded with unfilled resin in one hand and the light-curing tip in the other. On removal of the matrix she paints a thin layer of resin over the restoration and immediately light-cures it. This layer must be removed subsequently if etching and bonding materials are to be used.

Posterior composites

Pre-preparation

The pre-set tray is similar to that described for anterior composites but with the addition of matrix holders pre-loaded with a choice of matrix bands (clear, ultra-thin or annealed conventional metal ones) and a suitable selection of packing and shaping instruments specific to posterior composites.

Clinical procedure

- Etchant and bond are applied as described for anterior composites.
- The matrix band, flat plastic instrument and wedges are presented as described for amalgam restoration.
- Many operators prefer to burnish the contact point with a ball-ended instrument rather than a flat plastic one. In this case, the DA exchanges the plastic instrument for the burnisher by parallel exchange.
- Presentation of filling material. Posterior composite materials can be placed either directly

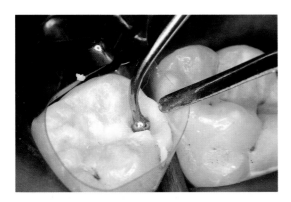

Figure 16.15

A posterior composite being packed while the DA holds the matrix tightly against the adjacent tooth, to maintain a good contact point.

from a pad and using hand instruments, or from a special amalgam carrier or a compule syringe. These should be handed to the dentist in the same way as for an amalgam carrier. If the dentist prefers to place the material directly from a pad by using a plastic instrument, the instrument is first directly placed in his right hand and the pad containing the material held as near as possible to the patient's mouth as described for placement of lining on pages 168–9.

- If a clear band is used, the maintenance of a good contact area can be facilitated by the DA holding the band against the adjacent tooth as each increment is placed (Figure 16.15). She must maintain this pressure while shining the light and curing the material. As each increment is subsequently placed, the DA moves the flat plastic instrument higher up towards the occlusal surface but continues to maintain firm contact of the band against the adjacent tooth.

- Posterior composite must be placed in increments. After placing each increment, the DA directly passes the packers and finally the occlusal shapers to the dentist. Some dentists prefer to use a tight cotton cylinder or pledget, moistened in bond to pack down the material, thus ensuring it is placed under maximum pressure. This is best achieved by placing the pledget in locking tweezers. The DA then moistens the ends of the pledget in bond and directly places the tweezers into the dentist's right hand, holding them at the extreme non-working end.

- Wedge and matrix-band removal and the checking of the occlusion are all as previously described for amalgam restoration.

- Finishing, with high-speed burs, finishing points or discs, is the same as described for anterior composites.

17 Prosthodontic procedures

Crown and bridge prosthodontics

Pre-preparation

The pre-set tray includes a block containing the burs and stones specific to the preparation of the type of crown or bridge, retraction cord, tweezers, cord-placement instrument, dental floss and a shade guide. A matching tub or two would contain impression and temporization materials with their respective syringes, mixing pads or slabs, and spatulas.

Clinical procedure

- The dentist administers local anaesthetic.
- While waiting for anaesthesia, the DA hands the dentist two different sizes of upper and lower trays for him to try. If study models are available, the DA can use these for measuring the trays. If no models are available, an experienced DA can usually gauge the approximate size of upper and lower trays needed.
- The DA coats the trays with the appropriate adhesive and sets them aside to dry.
- The impression syringe is assembled and made ready for use.
- The DA dispenses the appropriate amount of impression material(s) onto the mixing pad. If an auto-mixing system employing a cartridge and mixing tip is used, the appropriate cartridge is loaded into the gun and the corresponding tip fixed to the end.

This type of mixing system can be utilized in one of two ways. The material may be mixed and then dispensed from the mixing nozzle into the syringe and then into the impression tray. Alternatively,

some manufacturers provide a small injection tip which fits directly onto the mixing nozzle and this can then be used to syringe material *directly* into the preparation. This injection tip must then be removed to allow the DA to load material into the impression tray.

If the alginate-impression technique for making the temporary crown or bridge is to be used, an alginate impression of the appropriate arch is taken prior to beginning tooth preparation.

Preparation

The procedures for aspiration, soft-tissue retraction and cleansing of the preparation are similar to those described for an amalgam restoration (see page 168).

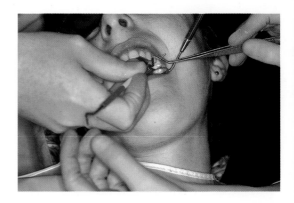

Figure 17.1

The DA holds the retraction cord in place while the dentist packs with the placement instrument in his right hand and holds the mirror with his left.

Pre-impression

The dentist places a cotton roll in the sulcus and dries the preparation while the DA picks up a pre-cut length of retraction cord with dressing tweezers held in her right hand and the cord-placement instrument in her left. She places the latter directly into the dentist's right hand and holds the retraction cord as close against the gingival margin as possible.

The cord is maintained in contact while the dentist packs it into the sulcus. This method allows the dentist to have both hands free to hold instruments. When packing into areas visible by direct vision, he can pack the first increment of cord and then, with a second placement instrument in his left hand to retain the cord in the sulcus, he may progressively pack in the next increment with the first instrument. This ensures that the cord does not spring out as he packs around the tooth margin. When packing on the lingual or palatal surface, he must use a mirror held in his left hand, with the placement instrument in his right (Figure 17.1).

If electrosurgery is used instead of retraction cord, the DA should fit the appropriate end into the electrosurgery handpiece and, holding it at its non-working end, place it directly into the dentist's right hand, locating the aspirator tip 'on site' and as close to the tooth as possible.

Impression

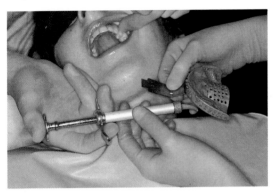

Figure 17.2

When the dentist signals that he is ready to take the impression, the DA mixes the impression material and loads it into both the injection syringe and the tray. The dentist removes the retraction cord with tweezers, discards both cord and instrument onto his right working surface and, if necessary, re-dries the preparation(s). The DA holds the syringe in her left hand and the loaded tray in her right and places the syringe directly into the dentist's right hand.

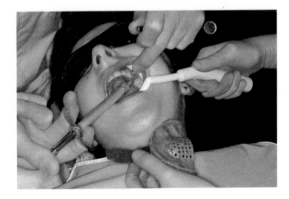

Figure 17.3

While the dentist is syringing the material, the DA transfers the loaded tray from her right to her left hand and picks up the aspirator with her right. This should be placed in the Fauces to aspirate saliva both for the patient's comfort and to keep the impression field dry. The aspirator must *not* be held on site because to do so would cause impression material to be aspirated up the tube causing a blockage in the system when it solidifies.

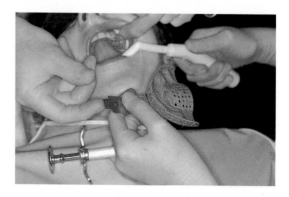

Figure 17.4

When the dentist has finished with the syringe, the DA takes it, grasping it in her little finger mid-way along its barrel, and places the loaded impression tray directly into the dentist's right hand.

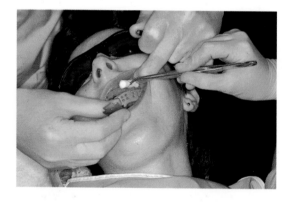

Figure 17.5

As the dentist places the tray into the mouth, but before it is fully seated, the DA puts down the aspirator tip, picks up a pair of dressing tweezers and, as the dentist retracts the lip with his left middle finger, she removes the cotton roll from the sulcus.

As soon as the dentist has seated the tray, and before replacing the aspirator in the patient's mouth, the DA must dismantle the impression syringe while the material within it is still soft.

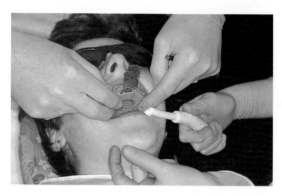

Figure 17.6

While the dentist holds the impression in place, the DA replaces the aspirator in the patient's mouth in the fauces position and maintains it here while the material is setting. This will remove accumulated saliva and contribute greatly to the patient's comfort. The DA maintains her left hand, finger and thumb open, in the transfer zone, ready to take back the impression after it has set.

When the material has set, the dentist removes the impression and the DA takes it in her left hand and places it in a dry plastic bag. She then mixes the opposing arch impression material, loads the tray and hands it to the dentist. It should be noted that the tray handle must be held as near to the tray as possible to give adequate length of handle for the dentist to grasp.

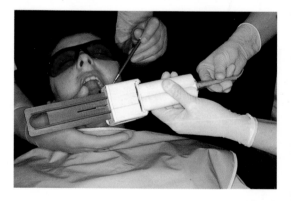

Figure 17.7

If an auto-mixing system is used to inject the impression material directly into the preparation, the whole mixing gun is handed to the dentist for him to hold in a palm grasp.

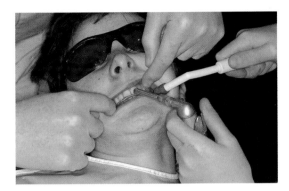

Figure 17.8

The occlusion has been registered with a wax wafer and the DA is cooling this with water spray, holding the aspirator on site to follow the syringe around the mouth.

Impression with reversible hydrocolloids

Pre-preparation

At the beginning of the week, the DA:

- Places enough tubes of tray and syringe material into the liquefying bath to last the week
- After the appropriate time, transfers the materials into the storage bath

Impression

The DA should:

- Select the correct size of tray and place stops if necessary
- Prepare the syringe by placing an 18-gauge needle in an anaesthetic syringe and bending the needle
- Connect the water-cooling tubes

- When the dentist indicates that he is ready to place the retraction cord, fill the tray with material
- Place the loaded tray in the tempering bath and press the timer
- Assist with the placement of retraction cord (see Figure 17.1)
- When the timer indicates that the material is ready, remove it and place gauze over the impression to absorb moisture
- Insert a cartridge of syringe material and hand it to the dentist
- While the dentist is syringing into the preparation, remove the gauze from the tray, connect the water-cooling tube and prepare to hand the tray to the dentist
- The impression procedure is then the same as that described earlier in the chapter

Occlusal registration

Wax wafer

The DA takes a small strip of wax, gently softens it in the bunsen flame and hands it to the dentist with her left hand. He places it over the arch and closes the patient's mouth in correct centric registration. While the dentist maintains the patient's mouth firmly closed, the DA chills the wax, holding the air–water syringe in her left hand and aspirator in the right to aspirate the coolant water (Figure 17.8). When the wax has hardened, the dentist takes the wafer out of the mouth and it is taken by the DA in her left hand.

Two-paste system in bite tray

The DA proportions and mixes the material, loads the bite tray and hands it to the dentist with her left hand. When the material is set, the tray is taken out of the mouth, received back by the DA in her left hand and placed carefully with the impression.

Face-bow registration

Whatever type of face-bow the dentist chooses to use, he should utilize the DA to help hold the bow and so make it far easier for him to manipulate it. In every case, the DA should load the bite fork with

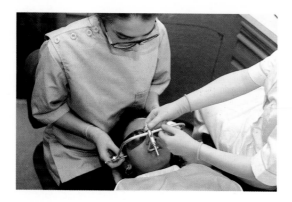

Figure 17.9

Face-bow registration. The dentist holds the face-bow in correct registration while the DA tightens the screws.

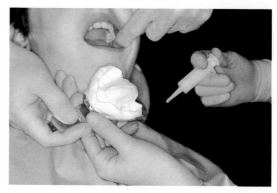

Figure 17.10

When temporization is required, the DA mixes the temporary material and, using the special syringe provided, places the material into the appropriate segment of the impression and places the loaded tray into the dentist's right hand for insertion into the mouth.

softened wax and hand it to the dentist for placement into the mouth. She may then chill the wax, using her air–water syringe and aspirator. She should then take hold of one side of the face-bow and hold it steady while the dentist places it onto the bite fork, and manipulates it into the correct position. Then, while the dentist holds the face-bow, the DA tightens the various locking devices (Figure 17.9). This procedure would be virtually impossible to do correctly without the assistance of a second pair of hands.

Temporization

Customized crown

Prior to beginning tooth preparation, an alginate impression of the appropriate arch is taken, removed, dried by the DA and set aside. Some dentists varnish the area of the impression corresponding to the preparations (Figures 17.10–17.14).

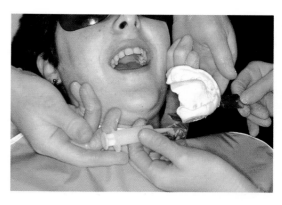

Figure 17.11

If the dentist prefers to syringe in the material himself, the DA places the alginate impression directly into his left hand and the syringe, holding it near the nozzle end, into his right.

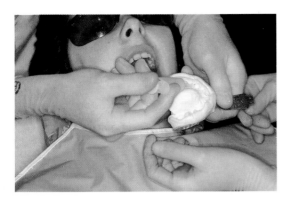

Figure 17.12

The dentist syringes the material into the impression. The DA holds her left hand ready to receive back the syringe.

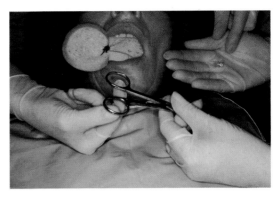

Figure 17.14

The DA places crown shears into the dentist's right hand, holding the celluloid crown form in her right palm.

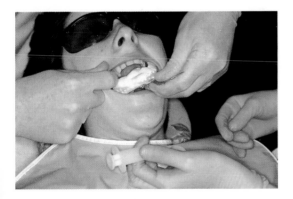

Figure 17.13

The DA takes away the empty syringe with her left hand, holding it between thumb and index finger but maintaining her hand in position ready to take back the tray.

When the material has set, she takes back the tray in her left palm. This procedure leaves her right hand free should she need to aspirate saliva while the tray is in the mouth.

Pre-formed metal, celluloid or polycarbonate crown

The DA can usually estimate the size of temporary crown needed. She first hands the dentist the protective sponge to place in position and then gives him the crown form to try in the mouth. If the celluloid type of form is used, the DA may trim the gingival contour of the crown form herself. However, if the dentist prefers to do this, the DA must hold the crown shears at their cutting end in her left hand, place them onto the dentist's right finger and thumb (Figure 17.14) and hold the crown form in her right palm. On completion of the trimming, the DA mixes the temporary material and loads it into the crown form.

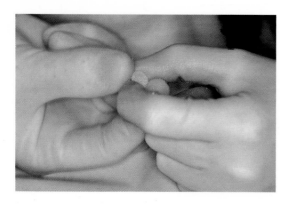

Figure 17.15

One of the problems in handling such a small object as a temporary crown is the difficulty of grasping it firmly in the correct position. This can be facilitated if the DA holds the crown so that the labio-lingual surface is free for the dentist to hold between his thumb and forefinger.

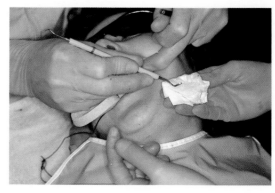

Figure 17.17

The dentist has trimmed away excess temporary cement. The DA wipes this from the instrument with a tissue.

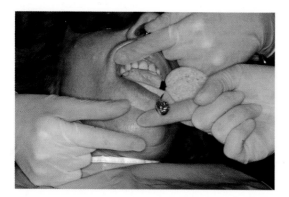

Figure 17.16

The DA can present a polycarbonate or metal molar crown form by placing it on the palmar surface of her finger, and delivering it to the dentist open side down with labio-lingual orientation towards him. He can then pick it up between his thumb and forefinger.

If a polycarbonate form is used, the dentist must trim this using a bur, usually in a straight handpiece. Both the appropriate handpiece and correct bur or stone would have been pre-set by a good DA.

Cementation of temporary crowns

After the dentist has placed a protective sponge in the patient's mouth and a cotton roll in the sulcus, the DA mixes the temporary cement, loads the crown and hands it to the dentist using one of the methods previously described.

Having seated the temporary crown onto the preparation, the DA passes a flat plastic or other trimming instrument to the dentist and picks up a folded tissue in her right hand, holding it between thumb and forefinger, as near to the preparation as possible. As the dentist trims the excess cement, he moves the trimming instrument just out of the mouth and the DA moves the tissue forwards and wipes the cement off the instrument (Figure 17.17).

Alternatively, the dentist may prefer to wait until the cement has set before removing the solidified pieces of excess cement with a suitable instrument. In this situation, the DA maintains the aspirator closely on site to remove the pieces. The advantage of maintaining the sponge in situ is that large pieces of dislodged cement will fall onto it instead of into the patient's mouth.

When the trimming is complete, the DA takes back the plastic instrument in her left hand, places the tissue and instrument on her work surface and exchanges them for occlusal registration paper. The occlusion is checked in the same way as that described for an amalgam restoration.

Shade selection

Ideally this should be done in natural daylight with the patient facing a window and either sitting upright or standing. However, in treatment areas with specially selected colour-matching ambient lighting, taking the shade with the patient supine may be equally effective.

Whichever method is used, the DA should stand or sit on the other side of the patient, holding the shade guide in her right hand, selecting individual tooth shades with her left and holding them near to the extreme end so that the dentist has sufficient length of holder to grasp. Many dentists like to have their DA's opinion on choice of shade.

Before dismissing the patient, the DA must fill out the laboratory card with the patient's name, type of restoration, shade, any special instructions and a return date. This date must then be communicated to the receptionist so that she can make an appointment which leaves sufficient time to take into account the interval required for the laboratory procedures. This can be done by giving the date on the treatment area to reception form (see page 37) sent with the patient. Alternatively, if the receptionist knows the working time required by the laboratory for each procedure, she may herself make the appointment and then fill in the return date on the laboratory card. In this case, the DA would leave the return date box on the card blank.

The information on the laboratory card—in particular the shade and date of return from the laboratory—should be duplicated onto the patient's record card. This ensures that a record is kept in case of lost laboratory cards and also provides a guide to the shade to be used in future work.

Try-in and cementation of permanent crown

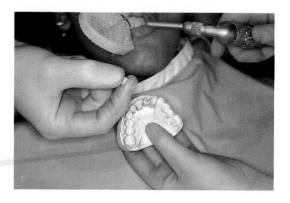

Figure 17.18

Before the dentist removes the temporary crown, the protective sponge must be positioned, after which the DA places into the dentist's right hand the instrument for removing the crown and holds the aspirator tip on site to retract the lip. When the dentist has removed the crown, the DA receives the instrument in her little finger and the discarded temporary crown in her palm. She places these on her work surface and discards the aspirator.

The DA picks up the model containing the permanent crown in her left hand and the air–water syringe in her right. By presenting the crown on the model, it is far easier for the dentist to pick it up to try in the mouth.

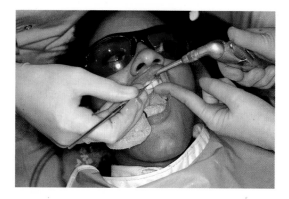

Figure 17.19

Having first dried the preparation, the DA holds the syringe on site to retract the lip. The dentist seats the crown and the DA holds it in place with her left index finger while he checks the marginal fit. This enables him to have both hands free to hold the probe and the mirror when checking the palatal or lingual margins. It is important for the DA to keep firm pressure on the crown to ensure it is properly seated.

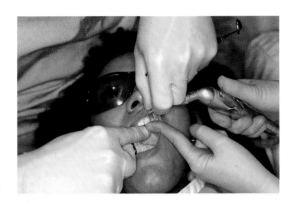

Figure 17.20

The DA then replaces her syringe and hands a length of dental floss to the dentist. This must be of sufficient length to wrap around his right and left middle fingers. The DA maintains firm pressure on the crown while the dentist flosses through the contact points to check these. Any adjustment can be made at this stage. Over-built contacts are often the cause of a crown not seating properly.

The dentist removes the crown, places it into the DA's left palm and, while she dries the inside of the crown, the dentist dries the preparation. If only a single syringe is available, then either the dentist or the DA will have to dry both crown *and* preparation.

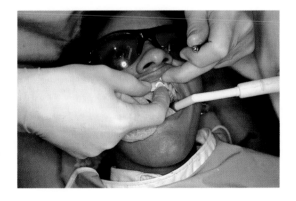

Figure 17.21

The DA mixes the luting cement, loads the crown and, holding it at its gingival end mesio-distally between her left thumb and index finger, hands it to the dentist so that he can grasp its lingual and labial surfaces between *his* right thumb and index finger.

The dentist seats the crown and maintains pressure with his right index finger while retracting the lip with his left index finger. The DA places the aspirator in the fauces position to evacuate fluids while the cement is setting.

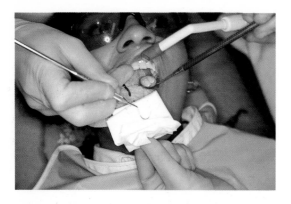

Figure 17.22

When the cement has set, the DA hands the dentist a flat plastic instrument or probe to remove excess cement. She then holds the aspirator on site to retract the lip. This gives perfect vision of the crown margins while leaving both the dentist's hands free, and also collects pieces of excess cement as the dentist removes them. The DA maintains a tissue in her left hand and wipes the tip of the instrument free of cement.

It is helpful to leave in the sponge at this stage so that any large pieces of cement fall onto the sponge and do not block the aspirator. Finally the occlusion is checked in the usual manner (as previously described).

Porcelain veneers

The increased use of porcelain veneers and the complex and critical techniques required for their correct placement requires the application of good teamwork between the dentist and his DA. If success if to be guaranteed, a systematic procedure must be strictly followed.

Pre-cementation preparation

Pre-cementation preparation of the veneer itself can be performed by the DA in accordance with the following procedure:

- A new pair of rubber gloves must be put on prior to handling the veneers.
- The veneers are placed into a suitable container or onto an adhesive palette, with labial surface facing downwards. The fitting surface is painted with conditioner, washed and dried. Dry bond is applied to ensure total drying.
- A suitable primer is painted on and the excess blown off with air from the air–water syringe.

Try-in and shading

Figure 17.23

The DA mixes trial shades of cementing medium. Most experienced DAs can make a fairly accurate judgment of the range of colours which may be required and can mix in shade modifiers where necessary. Several blends should be laid out on the pad and labelled with their constituent colours. The special instruments for coating veneers with luting medium are prepared. The dentist places the protective sponge in position.

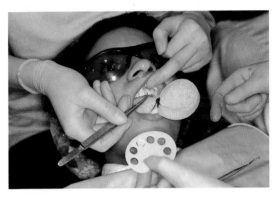

Figure 17.25

The dentist positions the first veneer.

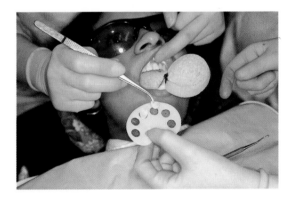

Figure 17.24

The DA loads each veneer with a trial shade. She places the container or palette holding the veneers between her left thumb and index finger, picks up a probe with her little finger and brings them to the transfer zone, holding them there. The dentist picks up the first veneer with the tweezers.

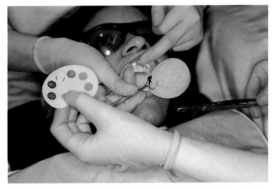

Figure 17.26

The DA takes away the tweezers with her right hand and raises her left to place the probe into the dentist's pen grasp.

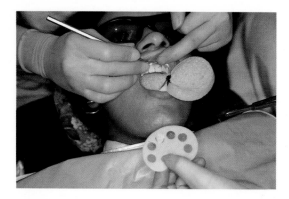

Figure 17.27

The dentist uses the probe to seat the veneer firmly, holding back the lip with his left middle finger while he checks the shade and fit.

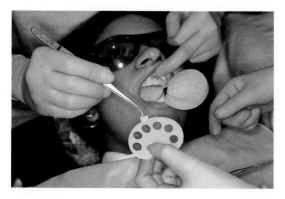

Figure 17.29

The dentist then picks up the second veneer and tries it on the next tooth, again checking fit and shade.

When fitting multiple veneers, it is important to try them on together to ensure that they all seat properly. Any adjustment can be made using a fine stone.

If the shade needs amending, the dentist removes the veneer, replaces it on the palette and the DA wipes off the composite with alcohol or acetone on a cotton bud. The DA places a new shade of composite on the veneers, replaces them on the palette and passes them back to the dentist for a retry.

When the correct shade match has been achieved, the DA must note the blend selected and wipe all the other blends off the mixing pad. The DA mixes a larger quantity of the material sufficient for final cementation of the veneer(s).

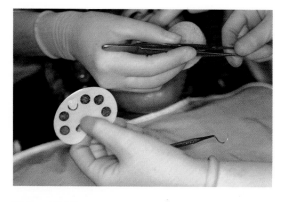

Figure 17.28

Still holding the palette in the transfer zone, the DA takes away the probe with her left little finger, replacing the tweezers directly into the dentist's right hand.

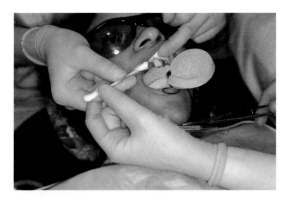

Figure 17.30

The dentist holds the veneer in place. Having taken away the probe with her little finger, the DA places a cotton bud directly in the dentist's right hand for him to wipe away excess material.

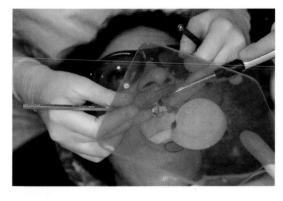

Figure 17.31

The dentist holds the veneer firmly in place while the DA cures the incisal one-third.

Cementation

Role of the dentist

- Pumices the surface of the teeth, washes and dries them
- Inserts soft metal separating strips between each of the teeth being treated
- Etches the appropriate enamel for 30 seconds and washes it off
- Inserts new cotton rolls and dries the tooth surface
- Paints the surface with a drying agent
- Paints the dry surface with a suitable bonding material containing a silane coupler

Role of the assistant

- Loads the veneer with the correct blend of composite cement
- Hands the palette containing the veneer to the dentist, who places the veneer on the tooth, seating it with a probe
- Removes the probe with her left little finger and exchanges it for a cotton bud or sable brush to remove excess material (Figure 17.30)
- Exchanges the cotton bud for the probe
- Cures the incisal one-third of the veneer while the dentist holds it firmly on the tooth with the probe—the dentist removes the remainder of the excess from the interproximal and incisal areas
- Cures the remainder of the surface of the veneer—the dentist must still maintain firm contact with the probe on the veneer (Figure 17.31)

Finishing

- Excess composite material around the periphery of the veneer is removed using 12- or 30-fluted burs or ultra-fine finishing diamonds and strips
- The DA hands floss to the dentist to check the contact points
- The occlusion is checked as described previously, taking particular care to check the protrusive and lateral excusions

Full and partial denture prostheses

Impressions

There is a common misconception that impressions (particularly of the maxillary arch) cannot be taken on patients lying totally supine because the gag reflex will be induced. A few simple precautions, however, can prevent any such occurrence and impressions of either arch, whether dentate or edentulous, and with any material, can be easily accomplished with total patient comfort.

The method of insertion described here causes the impression material to flow backwards and fill the space which the DA creates by making the bevel. In this way, the material flows only just past the post-dam border of the tray and will not be forced backwards to the patient's soft palate. Since the impression material does not contact the soft palate, the method described effectively prevents the gag reflex occurring.

It should be noted that this method places the *posterior* teeth into the material first, followed by the *anterior* teeth. The method most dentists use is to insert the tray in a direction such that the anterior teeth are placed into the impression material first, after which the posterior border of the tray is moved upwards. It is this technique which causes impression material to flow backwards towards the soft palate, producing large quantities of excess material which touch it and stimulate the gag reflex. This technique can be used for all types of impression materials and for both fixed and removable prostheses.

Clinical procedure

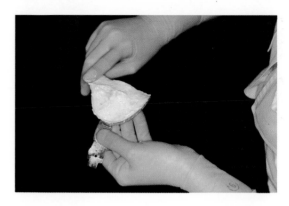

Figure 17.32

The DA loads the selected tray with the appropriate impression material. Immediately prior to handing the loaded tray to the dentist, she runs her right index finger across the post-dam border to wipe away material and create a positive 45° bevel.

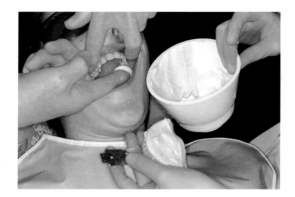

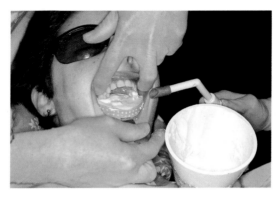

Figure 17.33

Holding the impression in her left hand and the bowl of excess impression material in her right, the DA has the loaded tray ready to place directly into the dentist's right hand and holds the bowl just to the left of the patient's chin.

Before the dentist inserts the tray, he scoops up a small quantity of material with his right index finger and places some in the palatal vault and over the occlusal surface of the teeth. This simple precaution results in a smooth impression, free of air bubbles. It is necessary to avoid such bubbles because they produce small pimples on the occlusal surface of the casting and so interfere with the precise seating of the models on each other. Similarly, in the edentulous mouth, material is placed first in the palatal vault and then into the sulcus adjacent to both tuberosities, prior to inserting the tray. This prevents entrapment of air in these critical areas, so producing a more accurate impression.

Figure 17.34

The dentist then inserts the tray, paying careful attention to the direction of insertion. The post-dam border is inserted first by directing the tray at about 45° to the palate. The DA transfers the bowl to her left hand and picks up the aspirator with her right.

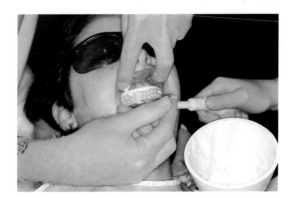

Figure 17.35

When this border is almost in contact with the posterior border of the palate, the dentist brings the anterior portion of the tray upwards, seats the entire impression and then performs any necessary muscle trimming. The DA inserts the aspirator tip in the left fauces to remove saliva for the patient's comfort.

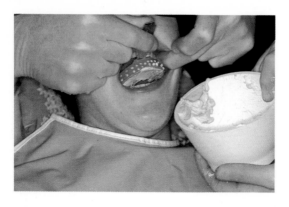

Figure 17.36

Lower impressions can be taken in a similar way but with the tray at 45° to the lower occlusal plane. The heels of the lower tray are placed onto the *molar* teeth first and the tray is then moved down over the anterior teeth.

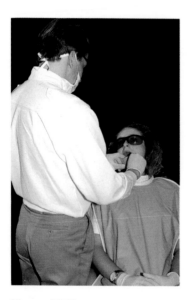

Figure 17.37

Occlusion registration with the dentist standing at 7 o'clock.

Occlusal registration

Preparation

A pre-set tray or tub should contain a vertical measuring device and marker, face-bow, wax rims on preliminary models, two wax knives, a bite plate, a bunsen burner, and shade and mould guides. For registration of the dentate patient, a separate tray with different colours of very thin registration paper should be prepared in appropriate holders together with appropriate burs and stones.

Clinical procedure

Measurement of the vertical height and jaw registration for the edentulous patient and of occlusal registration for the dentate patient can be achieved with the patient either sitting upright or supine. Authorities differ as to which method gives the more accurate registration. Some dentists find occlusal registration easiest to perform with the patient sitting upright. However, it must be remembered that the dentist can undergo body distortion in either the standing or the seated posture. To avoid this possibility, the five variables must be considered. Thus the patient's head should be vertical and rotated towards the dentist, who should stand in the 7 o'clock location facing the patient (Figure 17.37). Some authorities, however, maintain that accurate registration is not possible because the patient's head is rotated, which produces muscle imbalance. To avoid this, it is suggested that registration should be taken with the patient sitting upright and with the dentist standing directly behind the patient, which allows the patient to keep his head vertical.

However, if the dentist wishes to measure vertical height and occlusal registration while the patient is supine, there are two alternative approaches:

- From behind the patient with zero head tilt, zero rotation and the dentist seated in the 12 o'clock location (Figure 17.38). This is the method of choice.
- From the front of the patient by tilting the headrest forward to its maximum amount,

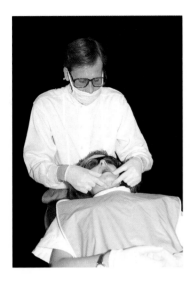

Figure 17.38

Occlusal registration with the dentist seated in the 12 o'clock location.

rotating the patient's head the full 45° towards the dentist, who sits in the 8 o'clock location facing the patient (Figure 17.39).

The DA heats the bite plate and levels the upper bite rim. When the dentist is satisfied that the correct upper occlusal plane has been established, the DA heats a wax knife, softens the lower rim and, while it is still on the model, hands it to the dentist. This provides a much easier method of transferring the rim, which the dentist can lift straight off the model. The DA holds the model in her left hand in the transfer zone and continues to heat the wax knife while the dentist makes the first trial registration of vertical height. He removes the lower rim and replaces it onto the model for the DA to resoften the surface.

When occlusal registration has been completed, the DA hands a chilled knife for the dentist to mark the centre and smile lines. She receives back the knife and presents the shade and mould guides to the dentist. The shade and mould should be entered not only on the laboratory sheet but also on the record card. This ensures that, should the laboratory lose the sheet, a record is available.

Try-in

The DA has the dentures ready on the model with a wax knife heated and available should the dentist need to remove teeth to make readjustments. When the dentist is satisfied that the occlusion is correct and the aesthetics to his satisfaction, the DA hands a large hand mirror to the patient so that he can view and give an opinion of the shade, aesthetics and tooth arrangement.

Fitting of dentures

The DA should place the finished dentures in a dish containing water ready to hand to the dentist and should have ready a straight handpiece with suitable trimming stone or bur in case this is needed for adjustments. The DA holds the bowl containing the dentures in the transfer zone. The dentist then takes them out of the bowl and inserts them into

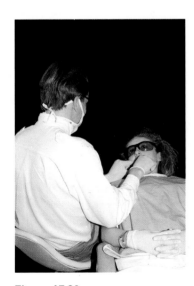

Figure 17.39

Occlusal registration from the front of the patient.

the patient's mouth. This method precludes the danger of dropping the dentures on the floor and damaging them.

During easing or trimming, the DA should blow air from the air–water syringe to remove acrylic debris and maintain clear vision for the dentist. Finally the occlusion is checked using registration paper in the same way as described on page 174.

18 Endodontic procedures

Cleaning and shaping

Pre-preparation

The tray should contain an 'endo' box with reamers and files arranged in sequence of use, X-ray films, paper points, irrigation syringe, fluid and a measuring device of choice. The pre-operative X-ray film should be mounted on the viewer. When the tooth is so badly broken down as to make placement of rubber dam difficult, the DA should present a copper or steel ring or temporary metal crown for the dentist to place, followed by a suitable cement to build up the crown.

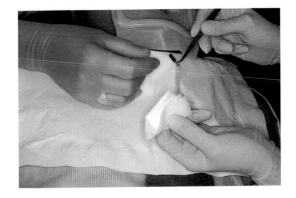

Clinical procedure

Figure 18.1

Rubber dam is placed and the access cavity prepared using the same four-handed technique described for cavity preparation (see pages 106–14). When access to the canal has been achieved, the DA takes the first file with dressing tweezers in her right hand, holding it at the junction of the handle and shaft, and takes a piece of folded gauze in her left hand. Pointing the base of the handle of the file towards the dentist's frontal plane, she places it directly into his right thumb and index finger. The dentist uses the file to remove vital pulp or necrotic tissue.

The DA then takes back the used file, holding it in the gauze, and makes ready a file with a stop fitted. She places this measured file into the dentist's fingers for him to take a diagnostic X-ray. The use of a folded gauze napkin prevents the possibility of the sharp and contaminated end of the file piercing the DA's glove and finger. Alternatively, instead of using gauze, a second pair of dressing tweezers may be used to take back the contaminated file.

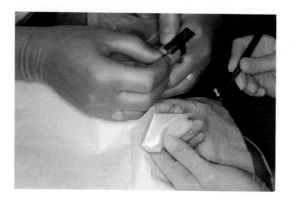

Figure 18.2

After the X-ray photograph has been taken, the DA holds the measuring device in her right hand and the gauze in her left. The dentist removes the diagnostic file from the tooth and measures it. Some endodontists prefer to have a measuring device mounted on their left hand and, in this case, the dentist would use this to make the measurement. The DA would then take it from him with the gauze in her left hand.

The DA then sets all the files at their correct working length in the 'endo' box, and picks up the first one in sequence with dressing tweezers in her right hand. Holding the file at the junction of the handle and shaft, she places it directly into the dentist's right hand (as in Figure 18.1) and holds her left hand in the transfer zone, ready to take back the file after use. While the dentist is shaping and cleaning the canal, she picks up the next file in sequence with the dressing tweezers and holds it in the transfer zone ready to present to the dentist.

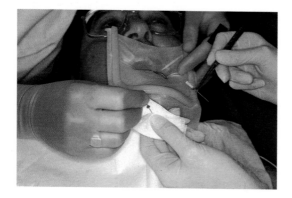

Figure 18.3

When he has finished with the first file, he removes it from the canal and the DA grasps the shaft in the napkin between her left thumb and index finger. As she takes it from the dentist, he keeps open his right thumb and index finger to allow her to place the second file from her right hand directly into his open fingers. It is interesting to note that this method is similar to the take and place method of exchanging hand instruments described on pages 126–7.

Between each filing, the canal(s) are irrigated. The DA holds the filled syringe in her left little finger to enable her to continue to hold the gauze with her thumb and index finger. She holds the aspirator with her right hand and aspirates while the dentist irrigates the canal. Cleaning and shaping is completed by repeating the entire process until all the sequential files are used.

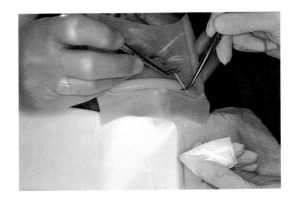

Figure 18.4

The DA hands a paper point to the dentist by holding it in her right hand using tweezers. He takes it, also using tweezers. The DA holds a tissue in her left hand, ready to receive back the used point. This technique ensures sterility of the points is maintained.

This way of working provides a very rapid and accurate method of cleaning root canals and guarantees that files are presented in the correct sequence and length.

If a giromatic type of handpiece is preferred to hand filing, the DA should place each measured file in sequence into the handpiece. The method used is identical to that described for bur exchange on pages 179–80, except that the file must be removed using tweezers to avoid puncture of the DA's glove by its sharp end.

Root filling

Pre-preparation

The tray should contain filling paste, spreaders and packers, irrigation syringe and fluid, paper points, measuring device and diagnostic X-ray film. The gutta percha points and tweezers are located separately on the dentist's side.

Clinical procedure

After placement of rubber dam, the temporary filling is removed. The access cavity is dried using the air–water syringe and then irrigated and dried with paper points.

The DA mixes the filling paste, and presents the pad and first packer or spreader in the transfer zone. Whilst the paste is being mixed, the dentist picks up the first point and measures it to correct length. He dips the point into the paste and inserts it into the canal. The DA takes the tweezers in her left hand and exchanges them for the packer or spreader by parallel exchange. When the first point is compacted, the DA takes back the packer, exchanges it for the tweezers and the dentist picks up the next point.

When root filling is completed, the DA helps with placement of a temporary seal, and removal of the rubber dam as described in earlier chapters. A post-operative X-ray is taken and the patient escorted from the treatment area.

19 Teaching four-handed dentistry

Dentists

The undergraduate teaching of correct work posture and assistant utilization varies widely from country to country and among different dental schools within each. A survey of the teaching of ergonomics completed in 1985 by the author for the Fédération Dentaire International showed that, outside the USA, the majority of dental schools had no organized program and that there were great discrepancies in the amount and scope of this teaching. Though the situation would seem to be improving slowly, there is as yet a failure to teach the principles of correct working posture and effective assistant utilization in the undergraduate curriculum as early and as comprehensively as is necessary. It is fully realized that there are financial constraints in many countries, but there is no doubt that a great deal more could still be done. It must be remembered that, on the whole, the operating techniques the undergraduate learns in dental school are what he takes with him into general practice. It becomes more difficult to change working methods following graduation.

Because of the inadequate teaching at undergraduate level, the graduate is launched into general practice with little or no idea of correct working posture, work simplification or team dentistry. It is not therefore surprising that the new dentist soon becomes accustomed to working in an incorrect posture and fails to utilize the DA properly. As a consequence, he soon starts to experience some of the pain and disabilities described in Chapter 6. Only a few, more motivated, graduates do try to remedy the omission by reference to textbooks and attendance at the occasional lecture or course.

Advantage should be taken of any postgraduate courses available on the subject. To achieve any benefit, such courses should be attended by the dental team—the dentist *and* his chairside DA— and should offer 'hands-on' participation. Attendance should be limited to a maximum number of 10 dentists with their DAs. Courses of this type run by the author have shown that in a single day both the principles and practical experience of correct working posture, patient seating, aspiration, soft-tissue control, mirror vision, tray systems and instrument handling can be taught to such a level as to enable participants to perform acceptable seated, team dentistry.

Dental assistants

To maximize the DA's effectiveness, she must not only be competent in practical skills but should also have a basic knowledge of dental theory related to those procedures she will encounter in general practice. There are several ways of achieving this:

- Full-time training courses
- Day release or evening classes
- In-service training

Full-time training courses

The ideal way is by attending a full-time training course in a dental or vocational training school. Because of the number of such schools in the USA, this is an excellent method of giving both practical and theoretical training to a comparatively large number of trainees. However, in the UK, vocational schools do not exist at present and full-time training is therefore limited to undergraduate dental schools where the intakes are extremely small.

Day release or evening classes

Working in general practice and attending day or evening classes is very effective but depends on the availability of such facilities in the area. A day-withdrawal type of class is preferable to an evening one because many trainees find it very onerous to attend after a full day's work. In the UK, the government-sponsored Youth Training Scheme is an excellent method of providing work experience in a general practice combined with a day in the classroom at a suitably accredited college.

In-service training

An alternative method of training is for the prospective DA to start as a junior—usually immediately on leaving school—in general practice. Though a high level of practical training can be achieved, it is more difficult for the trainee to learn the theory because the dentist can rarely find time in a busy working day to teach her. It is for this reason that the more motivated trainees eventually find it necessary to supplement their training with attendance at evening classes.

It is much more feasible for the new trainee to be taught the practical skills while working in practice. This should be the responsibility of a trained and experienced DA who might start by showing the workings of the various items of equipment and correct mixing of the basic materials used. The method most frequently employed, particularly in undergraduate teaching schools, is to provide the new trainee with a thick manual containing a very detailed, step-by-step list of all the procedures she will be expected to carry out. This tends to be learned parrot fashion and without any real understanding.

A better and more effective way is to limit the content to a list of the instruments and materials to make ready for each procedure. The actual chairside operative procedures are better taught using principles and rules. For example, by using models and illustrations, aspiration would be taught by giving the general principles which are outlined in Chapter 9 such as:

There are two basic positions of the tip, which are:
● On site, where soft-tissue retraction is required:
— The bevel is parallel to the tooth surface
— The tip is always on the side of the arch nearest to the DA
— It is placed 1 cm from the tooth
— It is level with its occlusal surface

● The fauces position, where no retraction is required

It is comparatively easy for a trainee to learn these simple rules, which can then be readily applied to any situation in the mouth.

After a very short time spent practising on another DA, the trainee should work with the dentist on patients as his principal chairside assistant but directly supervised by the senior DA. The dentist must schedule his appointments for the first day to allow for the extra time that will be required, since the trainee is obviously going to work much more slowly. Such time spent, however, will repay handsomely in the future because the level of skill of the trainee will be so much better.

Many dentists make the common mistake of believing that trainees can learn by standing and watching clinical procedures for days on end. In fact they learn very little of practical value in this way and quickly become disinterested and bored. Dentists also tend to underestimate the ability of even an inexperienced assistant to assimilate knowledge and acquire practical skills. For example it is possible to teach an untrained assistant within 10 minutes to perform, albeit slowly, an instrument-exchange technique such as parallel exchange.

Teaching instrument technique

The 'reverse presentation' technique should be used for every instrument and appliance (Figures 19.1–19.3). This technique gives the dentist the correct finger position for receiving the instrument while the DA has learned the correct presentation position and grasp for that instrument. Both should

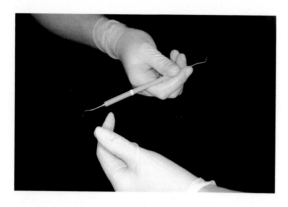

Figure 19.1

Reverse presentation technique
The dentist holds the instrument in precisely the grip he normally uses.

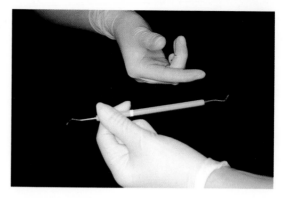

Figure 19.3

The DA takes the instrument from the dentist and both of their hands are kept in position. The dentist and DA are now able to take note of their respective finger and hand positions. This would be the presentation and receiving position for a hand instrument for the DA and the dentist respectively.

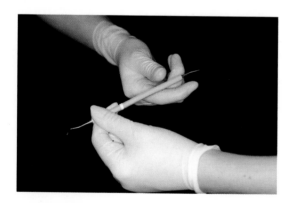

Figure 19.2

The DA grasps the non-working end of the instrument and the dentist releases his grasp but maintains his hand in the same position, with fingers open.

then memorize this and repeat the procedure several times, the DA alternately taking the instrument from the dentist and replacing it into his fingers. Many dentists are not aware of the grip or finger position which they use for instruments since it is usually a purely reflex one. In this way, individual operator variations are taken into account and the dentist and DA can then exchange any instrument or appliance smoothly and efficiently.

Finally, the principles propounded in this chapter may be summarized in the words of Benjamin Franklin, 'Tell me and I forget, show me and I remember, involve me and I learn.'

Reading list

ADA Council on Dental Materials, Dental Practice and Therapeutics, Infection control recommendations for the dental office, *JADA* (1988) **116**:241–8.

Altshuler, J L, Marketing cosmetic dentistry, *J Calif Dent Ass* (1989) **18**:8.

Altshuler J L, Johnson A, Manzoli N, The sixty second solution, *Dentistry* (1983) **3**:1.

Altshuler, J L, Romanowsky A, Instant photography: its application in the progressive dental office, *Dental Clinics of North America* (1970) **14**:2.

Blakeslee R W and Wolff M S, Infection control in the dental laboratory, *Quintessence Dent Technol* (1988) 141.

Boyd M A, Donaldson D, First year experience with a performance simulation system, *J Dent Educ* (1983) **47**:10.

Crowe C, Study underlines marketing value, *The Dentist* (1988) **6**:17.

Draycott A, Pilot survey of out-patient non-attendance, quoted in Woolgrove J, Cumberbatch G and Gelbier S, Increasing attendance by using personalised reminders, *Community Dental Health* (1988) **5**:389–93.

Editorial, Gloves, *Clinical Research Associates Newsletter* (1985) **9**:4.

Fédération Dentaire International, *Report of Working Group 3* (FDI: London 1985).

Goldstein R, *Change Your Smile* (Quintessence: Berlin 1988).

Holloway P M, Bucknell R A, Denton G W, *J Hosp Infection* (1986) **8**:39–46.

Ibsen R, *Smile Portfolio* (Den-Mat: Santa Maria, CA 1986).

Kilpatrick H, *Work Simplification in Dental Practice* (W B Saunders: Philadelphia 1979).

Koch R, *Mitt Reichsgessundh Amt* (1881) **1**:234.

Mandal A C, Work-chair with tilting seat, *Ergonomics* (1976) **19**:157–64.

Martin M, Letter to Editor: Glove-up advice, *The Dentist* (1988) **10**:11.

Molinari J, Gleason M, Cottore J et al, Comparison of dental surface disinfectants, *J Gen Dent* (May/June 1987).

O'Shea R M, Corah N L, Ayers W A, Sources of dentists' stress, *JADA* (1984) **109**:48.

Paul J E, Close-up on loupes, *The Dentist* (1988) **4**:30.

Paul J E, Influence of environment on the apprehensive patient, *Int Dent J* (1976) **25**:2.

Paul J E, *A Practical Guide to Assisted Operating* (BDA: London 1972).

Paul J E, Technical report no. 236: Survey on undergraduate teaching in dental ergonomics (Fédération Dentaire International, Commission on Dental Education and Practice: London 1985).

Paul J E, Posner B, *Developing the private sector in general practice* (Paul and Posner Seminars: Manchester 1987).

Powell M, Smith J W, Occupational stress in dentistry: the postural component, in *Proceedings of 2nd International Conference on Ergonomics, Dortmund* (Taylor and Francis: London 1964) 337–9.

Schön F, *Teamwork in the Dental Practice* (Quintessence: Berlin 1972).

Stombaugh F, Utilization of dental auxiliaries, *Quintessence International* (1979) **2**:17.

Turley M, Back pain and the dental student, *Quintessence International* (1983) **8**:1.

Wander P A, Gordon P D, *Dental Photography* (British Dental Association: London 1988).

Wilson G, Bacterial resistance, disinfection and

sterilization. In Wilson G, Miles A, Parker M T, eds, *Topley & Wilson Principles of Bacteriology, Virology and Immunity*, vol 1 (Edward Arnold: London 1984).

Wood P R, *The Dentist's Guide to Cross-Infection Control* (Update-Siebert: Guildford 1987).

Wood P R, Martin M V, The cost of cross-infection control, *Dental Practice* (1989) **27**:12–16.

Woolgrove J, Cumberbatch G, Gelbier S, Increasing attendance by using personalised reminders, *Community Dental Health* (1988) **5**:389–93.

Index

Page numbers in *italic* refer to illustrations

accountants, 59
addition silicone impressions, disinfection, 147
adhesive tape, colour coding with, 154
administration systems, computer, 60–2
advance appointments, 40
advertising, 14, 15
aerosols, cross-infection, 136
AIDS, 135
air conditioning, 8
air-water syringes:
    during examinations, 161
    removal of debris and saliva, 115
    removal of spray from mirrors, 112
    sterilization, 146
airway, protecting patient's, *94, 95*
alcohols, disinfecting with, 145
alginate impressions, disinfection, 147
alpha colour coding, filing systems, 43
alphabetical filing systems, 43
amalgam, procedures, 168, *169–75*
amalgam carriers, *122–3, 124*
American Dental Association, 16, 146, 147
anaesthesia, local, 20, 162–7, *162–7*
anterior teeth:
    composites, 177–82, *177–82*
    high-speed cutting, 101–3
antibiotics, 31
anticipation, work simplification, 150
antisepsis, 135
applications software, computers, 58–62
appointments, 29–42
    appointment books, 29–34, *32–3*
    appointment cards, 15–16, 25, 38–40
    buffer zones, 30, 31, 34
    date stamps, 42
    day sheets, 34
    with hygienists, 41–2
    making, 30–4
    methods of apportioning time, 36–7
    problems, 34–6
    recall systems, 40–1
aspirating syringes, 164
aspiration, 96–105, *97–105*
aspirators:
    disinfection, 140
    tubes, 96–9, *97–9*
autoclaves, 141–2, 152

Bacillus stearothermophilus, 143
back, seated posture, 69–77, *70–1, 73–6, 78*
back pain, 71–2, *72*, 75
back-projection film viewers, 13
back-up devices, computers, 56
background lighting, 6–7
bacteria, 135–6
banker's orders, 49
Beach, Dr Daryl, 72, 77
billing, fees, 50–1
biphenols, 145
bite-wing X-rays, 161–2, *161*
blinds, 7
blocks, bur, 150, *150*, 153
blood, cross-infection control, 135
    'blueprint', methods of apportioning time, 36–7
books:
    appointment books, 29–34, *32–3*
    patient information, 16
brick, internal decor, 4
bridge prosthodontics, 184–97, *184–97*
British Dental Health Foundation, 16
brochures:
    educational, 16
    practice, 13–14
Browne tubes, 141, *142–3*
buffer zones, appointments, 30, 31, 34
burs:
    blocks, 150, *150*, 153
    exchange of, 179–80
    ultrasonic cleaning, 140–1
    work simplification, 150

cameras, 17, *17*
Candida albicans, 136
cards see appointment cards; record cards
carpets, internal decor, 4
cash flow, 47
casts, models made from, 18
ceilings, internal decor, 4–5
cementation:
    glass-ionomer cements, 181–2, *181–2*
    permanent crowns, *192–4*
    porcelain veneers, 195–7, *197*
    temporary crowns, 191
Centers for Disease Control, 139
central processing units (CPUs), computers, 54

chairs:
    consultation area, 13
    operating stools, 85–6, *86*
    waiting areas, 9
    see also dental chairs
cheeks, control of, 106–8, *107*
chemical disinfection, 144–6
chemical sterilization, 143
chemiclave, 142
cheques, practice, 51
children:
    children's corners, 9
    crèches, 25
    marketing dentistry, 25
    seating in dental chair, 94
    videos, 18
chlorhexidine, 139, 145
chlorine, 145, 147
clamp holders, rubber dam, 157
clamps, rubber dam, 157, *158*
clinical examinations, 21–2
clinical systems, computer, 62
close-support technique, dental assistants, 88–95, *88–91*
clothing, cross-infection control, 148
clubs, dental health, 25
collection of fees, 47–51
colour-coding:
    bur blocks, 150, *150*
    filing systems, 43–5
    instruments, 153–4, *154*
    tray systems, 152, 153
colours:
    internal decor, 5, 9
    uniforms, 10
communication:
    between treatment area and reception, 37
    computer software, 59
    with ethnic groups, 26
    marketing dentistry, 12–18
    staff meetings, 27–8
complementary colour schemes, internal decor, 5
composites, procedures, 177–83, *177–83*
computers, 53–66
    hardware, 53–7, 62
    maintenance, 63–4, 65
    practice organization, 64
    purchase, 62–3
    recall systems, 40

computers (*cont*)
  software, 53, 57–62, 64
  training staff, 64–5
confirmation, treatment plans, 23–4
consultation appointments, 22–3
consultation area, 12–13
Cooper, K, 36
cord, retraction, *184*, 185
cork, internal decor, 4
corporate identity, 15
cosmetic dentistry, 11, 16
crèches, 25
credit cards, 19, 49
cross-infection control, 92, 135–48
crown prosthodontics, 184–97, *184–97*
curing lights, sterilization, 146, *146*
curtains, 7
custom-made appointment books, 30

daisywheel printers, 56
data storage, computers, 55
databases, computer software, 59–60
date stamps, 42
day release, dental assistants, 207
day sheets, 34
debris:
  cleaning instruments, 140
  mirror vision, 110
  removal of, 115
decor, practice image, 3–9
decor lighting, 7
deferred payments, 19
delivery grasp, instrument handling, 117–19
dental assistants:
  amalgam procedures, 168–76, *169–75*
  composite procedures, 177–83, *177–83*
  day sheets, 34
  duties, 91–5
  endodontic procedures, 203–5, *203–7*
  four-handed technique, 88–95, *88–91*
  instrument handling, 116–34, *117–33*
  learning instrument technique, 207–8, *208*
  maintenance of a clear operating field, 96–105, *97–105*
  maintenance of operating vision, 106–15, *107–15*
  photography, 17
  preparatory procedures, 157–67, *158–67*
  prosthodontic procedures, 184–202, *184–201*
  seated posture, *88–91*, 89–91
  training, 206–8
  work simplification, 149–54
dental chairs:
  dental assistant's posture, 90
  dentist's posture, 80–7, *82–6*
  seating the patient, 92–4, *93*

dental health clubs, 25
dental history, 21
dentists:
  amalgam procedures, 168–76, *169–75*
  composite procedures, 177–83, *177–83*
  communication with reception, 37
  endodontic procedures, 203–5, *203–7*
  exercise, 87
  four-handed technique, 88–95, *88–91*
  instrument handling, 116–34, *117–33*
  learning four-handed technique, 206, *208*
  maintenance of a clear operating field, 96–105, *97–105*
  maintenance of operating vision, 106–15, *107–15*
  preparatory procedures, 157–67, *158–67*
  prosthodontic procedures, 184–202, *184–201*
  relaxation, 34
  staff meetings, 27–8
  telephone calls, 34
  work simplification, 149–54
dentures:
  fitting, 201–2
  impressions, 198, *198–9*
  occlusal registration, 200–1, *200–1*
  try-in, 201
deposits, fees, 49
desks, consultation area, 13
desktop publishing, 58
despatching areas, dental laboratories, 148
diphenylalkane compounds, 145
discounts, on fees, 48–9
discs, vertebral, 71, 72
disinfection, 135, 138, 140, 144–6, 147
disk drives, computers, 55–6
disposable equipment, cross-infection control, 139–40
dot matrix printers, 56–7
dry-heat sterilization, 142
dry-zone technique, mirror vision, 111–12, *111*

education:
  children, 25
  communication, 12–18
  pamphlets, 9, 16
  patient, 9, 20
elderly patients, 25–6
electrosurgery, 185
emergencies, 27, 31
  buffer zone, 31, 34
  emergency trays, 152–3
endodontic instruments, ultrasonic cleaning, 140
endodontic procedures, 203–5, *203–5*
environment, 3–10, 26

estimations, methods of apportioning time, 36
ethanol, 145
ethnic groups, 26
evening classes, dental assistants, 207
examinations, 161, *161*
  clinical, 21–2
  preclinical, 21
  recall, 22
exchange of instruments, 126, *126–33*, 132–4
exercise, 87
extended payments, 49
external decor, 5
extraction forceps, handling, *125*
eye protection, 94–5, *94*

fabric wall-coverings, internal decor, 4
face-bow registration, 187–8, *188*
failed appointments, 35
fear of pain, 20
fees see payments
filing systems, 42–4
  computers, 59
finance charges, extended payments, 49
financial control, 45–52
'finger-control posture', 74–5, *75*
five variables, working posture, 78–81, *79*, 110
floors:
  disinfection, 138
  internal decor, 4
floss ligatures, 158
fluorescent lighting, 6, 7
formaldehyde, 142
four-handed techniques, 88–95, *88–91*
  teaching, 206–8, *208*
frames, rubber dam, 157
full-time training courses, dental assistants, 206
functional lighting, 6
fungi, 136

gagging, 84
gas sterilization, 147
glare, lighting, 6
glass-ionomer cements, 181–2, *181–2*
gloves, 138–9
gluteraldehyde, 138, 144, 147
graphics, computer software, 59
graphics cards, computers, 54–5

halogens, 145
handling instruments, 116–34, *117–33*
handpieces:
  sterilization, 146
  ultrasonic cleaning, 141
hands:
  gloves, 138–9
  washing, 139
hardware, computers, 53–7, 62

headphones, personal stereo systems, 8
heat-shrunk tubing, colour coding with, 154
heating, 8
hepatitis B (HBV), 135, 138–9, 140, 145
herpes, 136, 138
hexachlorophene, 145
high-volume evacuation, 96–105, *97–105*
HIV, 135
horizontal storage, record cards, 44
hourly rates, fee calculation, 45–7
hours, adapting practice hours, 20–1
hydrocolloid impressions, 187
  disinfection, 147
hygiene, cross-infection control, 92, 135–48
hygienists:
  appointments, 31, 41–2
  educating children, 25
  photography, 17
hypochlorite, 138

image, practice, 3–10
impressions:
  cross-infection control, 140, 146–8
  dentures, 198, *198–9*
  with reversible hydrocolloids, 187
  tub-tray system, 153
in-dwelling thermocouples, 143
in-service training, dental assistants, 207
infection, cross-infection control, 92, 135–48
infiltration, local anaesthesia, 165, *165*
injection techniques, local anaesthesia, 165, *165*
input units, computers, 54
instruments:
  colour-coding, 153–4, *154*
  disposable, 139–40
  handling, 116–34, *117–33*
  sterilization, 140–3, 146
  teaching instrument technique, 207–8, *208*
  tray systems, 151–4, *151*
  work simplification, 149–54
insurance schemes, 19
integrated high-volume evacuators, 99
internal decor, 3–9
intra-ligamentary injections, *164*, 167, *167*
introductory appointments, 34
iodine, 145
iodophores, 145, 147
isopropyl acetone, 142
isopropyl alcohol, 145

journal sheets, 51

keyboards, computers, 54

laboratories, cross-infection control, 146–8
language, ethnic groups, 26
laser printers, 56
late patients, 35
late running, buffer zone, 31
letters:
  computer-generated, *61*
  confirmation of treatment plan, 23–4
  word processors, 57
light curing tips, sterilization, 146, *146*
light pens, computers, 54
lighting, internal decor, 5–7, 9
lips, control of, 106–8, *107*, 110
local anaesthesia, 162–7, *162–7*
location, work simplification, 150–1
logos, 14–15, 40
loupes, magnifying, 86–7
louvre blinds, 7

magazines, 9
magnifying loupes, 86–7
mail-shots, practice brochures, 14
mailed appointments and reminders, 40–1
maintenance, computers, 63–4, 65
management *see* practice management
marketing, 11–28
  communication, 12–18
  market segmentation, 24–6
  planning treatment, 21–4
  staff-patient relationship, 26–7
masks, 138
medical histories:
  cross-infection control, 136–8
  forms, 21
meeting, staff, 27–8
memories, computers, 55
mental stress, 77
methylethyl ketone, 142
microprocessors, computers, 54
mirrors:
  handling, *121*
  mirror vision, 110–13, *111–13*
  specifications, 113–14, *114*
models:
  patient education, 18, *19*
  planning treatment with, 22
modems, computer, 57, 59
molars, high-speed cutting of left maxillary, 101, *102*
monitors, computers, 54
monochromatic colour schemes, internal decor, 5
mouse, computers, 54
mouth rinsing, 175–6
musculoskeletal pain, 69–71
music, 7–8

names, making appointments, 30
napkins, rubber dam, 158

needles:
  disposable, 139
  suturing, 139–40
nerve blocks, 166, *166*
networking, computers, 59
newsletters, 14
numerical filing systems, 43

obtuse-angled aspirator tubes, 97–9, *98–9*
occlusal registration:
  crowns and bridges, 187–8, *187–8*
  dentures, 200–1, *200–1*
one-write system, billing, 50–1
operating stools, 85–6, *86*
operating systems, computers, 57–8
'operator-to-reception' slips, 37, 50
oral thrush, 136
ordering, stock control, 52

pain:
  emergencies, 27, 31
  fear of, 20
  working postures, 69–71, 72, 75
paint, internal decor, 3
palm grasp, instrument handling, 117, *118*
palm-thumb grasp, instrument handling, 117, *118*
pamphlets, educational, 16
paper, internal decor, 3–4
parallel exchange, instruments, *128–31*
'parallel rule', working posture, 78, *78*
patients:
  appointment problems, 34–6
  cross-infection control, 136–8
  dentist's working posture, 78–87, *79–81*
  dismissal, 175–6
  education, 12–18, 20
  emergencies, 27, 31
  gagging, 84
  making appointments, 29–34, *32–3*
  payment facilities, 19–20
  planning treatment, 21–4
  preparation for treatment, 94–5, *94*
  reassurance, 20
  recall systems, 40–1
  seating, 92–4, *93*
  staff-patient relationship, 26–7
  telephone calls, 37–9
payments:
  collection of fees, 47–51
  estimates, 38
  failed appointments, 35
  fee calculation, 45–7
  financial control, 45–51
  methods of payment, 19–20, 48–9
  overdue fees, 31
  practice accounts, 51
pegboard transaction slips, 49, 50–1
pen grasp, instrument handling, 117, *118*

pen grip aspirator tubes, 96–7, *98*
periapical X-rays, 162
personal stereo systems, 8
phenols, 144–5
photography, 17–18
    tray system, 153
physical stress, 69–72, *70–1, 78*
planning:
    appointments, 37
    treatment, 21–4
    work simplification, 149
plastic filling instruments, handling, *120*
play areas, waiting rooms, 9
Polaroid photography, 17
poliomyelitis vaccination, 140
polishing, 179
polyether impressions, disinfection, 147
polysulfide impressions, disinfection, 147
porcelain veneers, 194–7, *195–7*
posterior composites, 182–3, *183*
posters, 16
posture:
    common faults, 81–5, *82–6*
    dental assistants, 88–91, *89–91*
    maintenance of correct posture, 78–
        81, *78–9*
    seated, 69–77, *70–1, 73–6*
    standing, 75
practice management:
    financial control, 45–52
    marketing, 11–28
    practice image, 3–10
    time management, 29–44
preclinical examinations, 21
preparatory procedures:
    examination, 161, *161*
    local anaesthesia, 162–7, *162–7*
    rubber dam, 157–8, *158–60*
    X-rays, 161–2, *161*
presents, for children, 25
printers, computer, 56–7
private patients, fee calculation, 45–7
probes, handling, *121*
production areas, dental laboratories,
    147–8
prosthodontic procedures, 184–202,
    184–201
punches, rubber dam, 157

quarternary ammonium compounds,
    145–6
questionnaires, telephone, 38–9

racks, tray systems, 152
reassurance, patients, 20
recall examinations, 22
recall systems, 40–1
receiving areas, dental laboratories, 147
reception areas, 8
receptionists, 8, 27
    clothing, 10

receptionists (*cont*)
    collection of fees, 47–8, 49–51
    communication with dentists, 37
    day sheets, 34
    making appointments, 29, 35, 37
    telephones, 37–9
record cards:
    date stamping, 42
    filing, 42–4
    recording payments on, 49
    storage, 44
records, computer, 59–60, 61–2
relational databases, 60
relaxation, dentists, 34
reminders:
    for children, 25
    recall systems, 40–1
    telephone calls, 35
resin, composite, 182
restorative procedures:
    amalgam. 168, *169–75*
    composites, 177–83, *177–83*
retraction cord, *184*, 185
reverse palm-thumb grasp, instrument
    handling, 97, *98*, 117
'reverse presentation' technique,
    instruments, 207–8, *208*
reversible hydrocolloid impressions, 187
rewards, for children, 25
rinsing, mouth, 175–6
root filling, *204–5*, 205
rotary files, record cards, 44
rotary instruments:
    blocks, 153
    exchange of burs, 179–80
rubber dam, 157–8, *158–60*, 177

saliva:
    cross-infection control, 135
    removal of, 115
scanners, computers, 54
seated posture, 69–77, *70–1, 73–6*
    common faults, 81–5, *82–6*
    dental assistants, 88–91, *98–91*
    maintenance of correct posture, 78–
        81, *78–9*
seating *see* chairs
security, computer data, 64
shade selection, crowns, 191
shaving cream, 158
silicone rubber, colour coding with, 154
simplification, work, 149–54
sodium hypochlorite, 145
soft-tissue control, 106–10, *107–9*
software, computers, 53, 57–62, 64
spectacles, protective, 94–5, *94*, 138
spine, seated posture, 69–77, *70–1,
    73–6, 78*
spitoons, disinfection, 140
splatter, cross-infection, 136
sponges, protecting the airway, *94, 95*

spore strips, 143
spores:
    bacterial, 135–6
    fungi, 136
spray, mirror vision, 110–13, *113*
spreadsheets, computer software, 58–9
staff:
    computer training, 64–5
    cross-infection control, 140
    meetings, 27–8
    staff-patient relationship, 26–7
    vaccination, 140
    see also dental assistants: dentists;
        hygienists; receptionists
stamps:
    date, 42
    rubber dam, 157
standardization, work simplification, 150
standing orders, 19, 49
standing posture, 75
stationery, 14–16
sterilization, 135
    connected instruments, 146
    in dental laboratories, 147
    procedures, 140–3
    tray systems, 151–2
stock control, 51–2
stools:
    dental assistants, 91
    operating, 85–6, *86*
storage:
    computers, 55
    record cards, 44
    tray systems, 152
stress:
    mental, 77
    physical, 69–72, *70–1, 78*
suction, 96–105, *97–105*, 138
summaries, treatment, 50
surface anaesthesia, 162, *162*
surfaces, disinfection, 138
surfactants, mirror vision, 112–13, *113*
suturing needles, 139–40
swapped appointments, 36
syringes, local anaesthesia, 162–4, *162–4*

T-cards, stock control, 51–2
tabs, filing systems, 44
tape, colour coding with, 154
teaching four-handed technique, 206–8,
    208
technicians:
    cross-infection control, 146–8
    date sheets and, 34
telephones:
    communication between treatment
        area and reception, 37
    computer modems, 57
    dentist's calls, 34
    failed appointments, 35
    patients' phone numbers, 30

telephones (*cont*)
    questionnaires, 38–9
    recall systems, 35, 40
    receptionists and, 37–9
    staff-patient relationships, 27
telescopic loupes, 86
temperature control, 8
temporization, crowns, 188–91, *188–90*
tetanus vaccination, 140
textures, internal decor, 3–5, 9
thermocouples, in-dwelling, 143
thrush, 136
time, appointments, 30–1
time management:
    appointment books, 29–34, *32–3*
    filing systems, 42–4
    methods of apportioning time, 36–7
    problems in appointment-making, 34–6
    recall systems, 41–2
time management appointment system, 29
time-steam-temperature (TST) strips, 141, 142–3, *143*
tongue, control of, 106, 107–10, *107–9*
toys, children's corners, 9
training:
    cross-infection control, 140
    dental assistants, 206–8
transaction slips, billing, 49, 50–1
transfer techniques, instrument handling, *118–25*, 119–25
'transfer zone', instrument handling, 116, *117*
tray systems, 149
    for composite restorations, 177, *177*, 182

tray systems (*cont*)
    cross-infection control, 138
    for crown and bridge prosthodontics, 184
    design, 151–2
    for endodontic procedures, 203
    planning, 152–3
    setting a tray, 153
    storage, 152
    tub-tray system, 153
    work simplification, 151–4, *151*
treatment:
    appointments, 31
    planning, 21–4
    summaries, 50
treatment area, preparation of, 92
'trigger' cards, 16
tub-tray system, 153
tuberculosis vaccination, 140
tungsten lighting, 6–7
tweezers, handling, *121*

ultra-short appointments, 31
ultrasonic cleaning, 140–1
uniforms, 9–10, 148
United States Environmental Protection Agency, 143
updating service, 18–19

vaccination, 140
varnish:
    colour coding with, 154
    glass-ionomer cements, 181–2, *182*
veneers, porcelain, 194–7, *195–7*
Venetian blinds, 7
verbal communication, 12–13, 37

vertebrae, 71, 72
vertical storage, records cards, 44
video graphics array (VGA) systems, 55
videos, 9, 18
viruses, 136
    computer, 63
visual communication, 17–18
visual display units/terminals (VDU/Ts), 54
visual foci, 7

waiting areas, 8–9
    children's corners, 9
    decor, 3–5, 7
    lighting, 7
walls, internal decor, 3–4
washing hands, 139
wax wafers, occlusal registration, 187, *187*
wetting agents, mirror vision, 112–13, *113*
windows, 7
wipes, disinfectant, 145
wood, internal decor, 4
wordprocessors, 24, 57, 58, 63
work simplification, 149–54
written communication, 13–15, 23–4, 37

X-rays, 13, 21
    disinfection of packets, 140
    endodontic procedures, 203
    X-ray procedures, 161, *161*

Youth Training Scheme, 207

zoning system, cross-infection control, 138